Asa's Story

Asa's Story

A Child's Struggle
A Family's Victory
Against All Odds

GUNNAR OHRLANDER

NEW HORIZON PRESS
Far Hills, New Jersey

This translated edition of the Swedish original title "Asa's Journal" is published by agreement with Bra Böcker Publishing Group, Höganäs, Sweden.

Translated into English by Patrick Smith.

Library of Congress Catalog Card Number: 91-53080
Gunnar Ohrlander
Asa's Story
ISBN: 0-88282-041-9
New Horizon Press

Acknowledgment

The author wishes particularly to thank The Research Council for contributing financially to the studies carried out as a basis for this book and to thank the physiotherapists and the doctors who have elucidated the casebook studies and checked facts.

PART ONE

Chapter One

I've fetched in the rabbit from the garden. She's sitting in front of me on the desk. She sits quite still. Sometimes she opens out her ears and listens to the sounds of our house.

Daddy puffs and blows when he sleeps. Mummy lies quietly beside him. She's rather small and chubby—soft and white as a bun before it's put in the oven. My twin sister Berit sleeps on the first floor in our house. Berit's sensible, successful, and beautiful. She gets top marks in everything. At night she grinds her teeth.

The other children, those who were children when my story begins, have already left home.

Soon it will be midnight. The yellow light from the lamp rains down over the desk. I listen to the sounds of the sleeping house and, behind them, to the silence. In the silence there's a story. I sit as still as the rabbit and let the story approach.

If they knew what I was up to now! If they knew they'd gather round me, they'd squint at the papers on the desk, and Mummy would ask in her brightest voice: Why are you sitting here, Asa? What is it you want to talk about?

They think one must have a reason. They'd destroy the story. They'd begin to wonder and behind their wondering I'd hear the other questions, their uneasiness about what happened: You think what we did was wrong, Asa?

Autumn breathes outside my window. People huddle up and whimper in their sleep about what they've done and what they haven't done. Fifteen years have passed. There are things I remember. Pictures drift by like light buoys. I cling to a small gym mat. I can still hear the cries. I know now the cries are mine.

We travelled into darkness. That's what I want to talk about, that journey into darkness. And to talk about it I have to make it again.

They said we travelled together. But we didn't. They travelled and they dragged me after them. They kept saying we'd find our way out. Out of the darkness. If I hadn't been so close to screaming myself to death I might have laughed myself to death. I didn't know what they were after. Children can't think like that, not children as small as I was. I was eight months when they started. Eight months and thirteen days.

I see the gym mat clearly. I lie on the mat. I lie on it for days, for months. The mat is stuffed with something soft and it's covered with plastic. One side of it is green, the other is red. The mat is still there. It's in the garden. I use it to protect my rabbit hutch. That's where the rabbit lives. She sits there and sniffs with her damp nose and looks at me with her black eyes.

They were travelling into darkness to find the light. It was a time when everything seemed possible. Everything good and everything bad. All over the world people lived as though intoxicated with hope. On the other hand, maybe that's the sort of thing they said afterwards.

How is one to find light in darkness? The idea seems ridiculous. Sensible people keep away from ideas like that. You don't travel into the desert to look for water. And if you set off into the darkness—if you really travel into it—you don't come back.

We didn't intend to come back, Daddy says. That wasn't what we were after. We wanted to find something new. Beyond the darkness and out on the other side.

There's nothing to find on the other side, I could have told him that. There is no other side. Only darkness. I'd have told him that if I'd been able to.

But I couldn't talk. I could only scream. First I screamed

my own scream. That's the scream I can still hear. When it came to an end, I screamed the scream all children scream. The darkness they decided to travel into was my darkness. It was my brain, the brain of a child. They thought they could create light in there the way alchemists long ago thought they could create gold.

What sort of arrogance drove them on? We know nothing, almost nothing about the brain. How can human beings understand the human brain? It sounds odd. It *is* odd. The brain understanding the brain!

At the precise point where tiny currents of energy in the brain become thoughts and consciousness: that's where God is. So it says on a piece of paper I've saved.

Once upon a time man stood at the edge of the ocean and looked out over the water. And he saw the curve of the ocean. He wondered about the snake on the other side, the snake lying in the water and holding all the world together. Man intended to find the snake.

But there was no snake out there. There was only more sea and land. And when man had finished travelling, he found himself back where he started.

Man pointed his telescopes out at space. Even then—and it was a very long time ago—wise men knew more about space than man now knows about the brain.

And they were going to travel into the brain. My brain!

You don't believe this of course. You say I'm lying. And my answer is: Of course I'm lying! My life then is a clock that's fallen on the floor. The pieces are scattered everywhere. I must recreate the pieces that are missing.

After all, I remember almost nothing. Only how it felt, and the plastic mat. I have the notes, the documents others kept. I have the case history from the hospital. Daddy keeps it at the bottom of one of his drawers. There are gaps everywhere. It's like looking into the mouth of a child just cutting its second teeth.

Do I sometimes sound sensible about all this? If I do, it's stolen wisdom—wisdom I've taken from others. The world is full of good sense, Daddy says. The sensible people have taken over. That's why the world looks the way it does.

Daddy narrows his eyes and purses his lips when he says this. He looks crafty when he says it. It's quite a while since anyone cared about what he says.

At first I cried because of all the gaps. Everything was a mess. Evening after evening I've sat here with my rabbit and listened to the story of what happened that time fifteen years ago. To the story of their journey into me, of the doctor from Prague and of how conflicting systems converged inside me. The desk is full of bits and pieces, papers and records. I'll put together what I have. The rest I'll have to make up as I go along.

I've read about expeditions. About men who travelled to the South Pole with sledges and huge snow shoes. They packed their bags with warm underclothes, woolen mittens, thermoses, and sandwiches. Their wives and children stood on the shore at home and waved goodbye. And off the men went, out into the unknown.

That's how I'd like to think of the expedition into my brain. As an old-fashioned expedition. With Daddy wearing heavy boots and trousers that can stand up to tough going. And a rucksack, with ropes and grappling-irons hanging from it. And Mummy checking the emergency supplies. She has to go back at the last minute to make sure all the doors are locked.

Daddy gets angry and tramps around in circles. He says: Of course Mummy hasn't forgotten anything. In any case, nothing they can carry with them. But that's the fate of modern women, he says. They act like farmers' wives who keep the keys in their apron pocket and make sure the last thing they do is lock the larder door. Only there aren't any larders anymore. Mummy searches and Daddy scrapes his feet angrily through the sand outside the house. Mummy's searching for a life women lived a long time ago.

Daddy often gets angry when there's no reason to.

And so they set off. They were going to outdo the explorers who discovered the South Pole. They were going to travel farther than the planet that burned in Galileo's eye. They travelled beyond the Milky Way and right into my brain. In there they made their way through dark landscapes, listening and reconnoitering. They were searching for tracks made once upon a time when life began. They were going back to the time when the earth still puffed and sweated fiery lava and when the fish of the sea began to breathe.

It's all in there in the child's brain, they said. You can hear the fish breathe in there. In there the lizards crawl and cry against the old, burning skies.

They were going to find the secrets of our species and make my brain do what evolution had intended it for. The brain is built up of all life that has been lived. The brain is everything evolution has led to. The brain is like the sea beds.

I was going to have to do what I was incapable of doing. I was going to creep like a lizard, turn like a baby ape, and stand up on my own two feet.

I screamed. My anguish was as old as the lizards they talked of. With their heavy boots they tramped across fragile structures and broke pieces off and hacked their way through and set up camp in a landscape no one has the right to enter. Leave me alone! That was what my cries meant. There's nothing to understand! You're fooling yourselves. The number of brain cells—so it says on another scrap of paper—is beyond human understanding. There are more brain cells than there are crawling things in all the ant hills in the country. Anyone who sets about counting the number of cells in a single brain will need hundreds of years.

It was on the small red-green mat that their expedition took place. Everything happened on that mat. I saw Daddy's shadow. He lay on top of me. All eighty kilos of him pressed me down against the mat. He held me and made sure I had the little round wooden stick in my hand. A red stick. It's still in my desk drawer.

Daddy muttered and grunted with the effort. He said things to overcome some of the anxiety. He said: Asa's a fighter. Asa's objecting. That's good! We're going to do the impossible. Mummy's face was blotchy with nervousness and tension. The idea was that I was to scream myself up on all fours. I was to object until I overturned. Over and up and start crawling!

But I couldn't. I couldn't crawl. I didn't want to crawl!

§

A warm autumn. At midnight it's still nudging in heat across the window sill. The rabbit in front of me sniffs towards the window. Out there the air lies like a blanket, damp with a thousand tiny drops after today's rain. The yellow arc lamps from the motorway strike upwards and the light remains suspended as though a huge roof had been thrown across the sky.

My story begins in Prague.

Several years before I was born it's already there, my beginning, with a doctor working in the pediatric clinic. He must be old now, probably over eighty.

If only I'd known then he was the one behind it all. I'd have bitten him with my first teeth.

They've spoken of him, the doctor with the funny name. I used to think of him as a thin man with thin black hair. I thought of his hair plastered down in black stripes across his forehead. I thought of his bony fingers and rigid eyes.

When the doctor comes the children hide.

He's a man of principle, as my talented sister Berit would have said. Berit knows a lot of words.

But, anyway, he's not like that. Not in the least. So Daddy says. The doctor has kind, brown eyes. He spreads love around him. He's like a warm lamp.

They talk about the doctor as though he were Jesus.

They talk about the sadness behind his friendly gaze. The sadness over countries where people are always cold and the sadness over children who can't walk.

Daddy takes out his big album with photographs and pictures he cut out of newspapers. He does it several times a year and he riffles through the pictures from Prague. He talks about the spring in Prague, about the water that once ran faster under the bridges and about a mountain he calls the White Mountain where, he says, a famous battle once took place.

In fact he's raving, because he's never been to Prague. Nor has he ever met the doctor. He raves and he defends what they did.

In one photo I see a lorry. Young Czechs are standing on the platform. They're holding the Czech flag spread out above their heads. Mummy's eyes become big and heavy when she looks at the picture. I can see from her eyes that she's on the verge of tears.

At that time the doctor worked at the pediatric clinic at the university in Prague. He'd been banished for a while. He wasn't permitted to work at the university. There were students there and the doctor wasn't good for students. He was religious.

A Catholic, Mummy says.

He didn't hide it. In his lectures he smuggled his faith across the boundaries that had been set up. He was forbidden to work in Prague.

Good, I say.

Be quiet, Daddy says.

Why should I be quiet? They're always babbling about how the Church is wrong. It's wrong to believe in God. There's no God and there are no ghosts. They're not being consistent. Nothing about them is really consistent. Now suddenly a doctor who was a Catholic was fine.

You don't understand that sort of thing, Daddy says.

That's what he usually says when he can't find an answer.

Spring came to Prague. The doctor returned. Mummy talks about longing. People were outdoors all the time. They were out on the streets, their doors stood wide open. The doctor returned.

The time had come, Daddy said.

Everything was going to happen and it would all happen at the same time. The spring made people heady and they pushed their excitement in front of them. The world waited, hoped, worried.

The doctor worked like a madman. There were children who couldn't walk. So many of them! The doctor had found out things no one else knew about. The doctor was going to teach the crippled children to walk.

Mummy and Daddy say it's all connected. With me. Far away in a worn-out Europe, soiled with coal smoke, there was a doctor who worked for the birth of what was new.

§

I was what was new. Daddy's glued the pictures beside each other in the big album. The picture of the young Czechs on the lorry and the picture of the place where I was made. Daddy sits with the pictures in front of him and he's quiet for a long time. He says he's listening to the pictures. He says there are similarities.

But the pictures are separated by several years. One of them shows a river far up in the north of Sweden flowing between steep banks. The photo is blurred. In one corner you can just make out an old railway station. It was there, outside the station building, that I was made.

I try to imagine Daddy as he was then. He's rather thin and a little round-shouldered. His face and his pointed nose make you think of dreams that were smashed to pieces. He rattles north in an old Peugeot Combi with jerry cans full of fuel oil and with music from the stereo. In those days people used fuel oil instead of diesel oil in their cars. He smiles. He's back up there somewhere at the North Pole.

There was no tax on fuel oil. People could drive a thousand kilometres for twenty crowns.

He drives along the river up there in the north, thousands of kilometres from Prague. He's on his way to liberate the people. He had a bee in his bonnet about liberating people. Everywhere he went he was going to liberate them: lumberjacks, peasants, railway workers. Behind him comes the motorcade with the Rabble. That was what he called them. They were actors and actresses he'd enticed into following him and they came with their children, their children's grandmothers, theater scenery, lamps and technicians.

They swarmed into the village by the river. Soon it was all a mess, like most things Mummy and Daddy are connected with.

I wrote a play, Daddy says, and makes a mark with a pen on the photograph. There, behind that window, I wrote a play.

He talks about lumberjacks and log-drivers who smelled of engine oil and snuff. He collected words for his play from the forests, he hacked them off the way bark is hacked off timber. Suddenly he's beaming and the story takes off.

The people living at the North Pole were going to be moved south. That was what had been decided. But they didn't want to move. They stayed where they were up at their North Pole and held on. I don't know why. They were happy amongst the mosquitoes. The temperature dropped to forty degrees below freezing in winter.

Yet they liked being there. The play was a success. People came from all over the North Pole. They came on tractors and brought their own chairs to make sure of getting a seat at Daddy's theater.

The papers wrote that Daddy was political.

Maoist, Mummy says.

Whatever that is. They'd read a book written by a fat Chinaman who had a wart on his face.

We were Maoists, Mummy says.

My aunt has a cat called Mao. My aunt was also a Maoist. When everyone forgot the fat Chinaman, she called her cat after him.

I think it seems odd. They talk about things I don't think existed. Not that way, anyway. Daddy rattled out of the forest in his Peugeot, and now that I've become older and wiser, I know what the forest was called. Its real name was Sherwood Forest.

I know almost everything about Sherwood Forest. When Daddy read a book about Robin Hood it was really Daddy who came riding with Friar Tuck and all the others to save people and liberate them and shoot off their arrows. There were no fat Chinamen in Sherwood Forest. They've made that up. Like other things they talk about. I don't say that to him because he might be hurt. Daddy says he's telling the truth. Dreams are true.

§

And so is the tale about the two nights.

The Rabble put on Daddy's play in the village by the river. When it was over, and people had cheered and cried and signed appeals, the Rabble made their way home towards the closed-down railway station. Mummy and Daddy floated. Like everything else. That's because of the northern light. Those who have once walked with light in their hair up there are never the same again, Daddy says. It was in the middle of the night, but the light was there just the same. Daddy's voice thickens when he talks about it. He blows his nose and takes out maps to show the places with the funny names.

Here's the river! And Morjärv and, far to the east, Jouksengi. There, in the forest on the ridge above Jouksengi, they lived a whole summer and listened at night to the horses running along the village road.

Further up along the river comes Överkalix. You can see the church from far away and it seems like the church and the houses are floating out on the water. The light shimmers over the roofs. This light is everywhere! The air splits and you think you see a mirage, a town that floats and is reflected upside down.

Mummy and Daddy were in love and knew that if this evening was possible, so was everything else. Daddy talks about how he felt that time. He talks about man's liberation. It sounds high-faluting. He falls silent and his face becomes red. You can see he liked big words once upon a time.

All that bright night the party went on in the village. The Rabble sang, the lumberjacks and peasants laughed and drank. They said Sweden's power comes from our rivers. We'll turn off the switch! The lights will go out in the Palace in Stockholm! The time has come!

They talked about courage and fighting spirit. And while the night was still filled with its strange light, they staggered around in the forest. They kept their Forest Brew fermenting in the heat of the anthills. Right there in the anthill were glass containers with a dreadful mixture of water, sugar, and yeast. And further in, behind the undergrowth, you could find cold springs where bottles of moonshine *schnapps* they called Forest Star had been hidden to keep them cold.

Mummy put her arms around Daddy. I can see them standing there, hugging and stumbling and falling in the soft grass that no one bothers to cut anymore. A child! I don't know which of them said it first. Out of all that is best, freedom, a new world, new human beings—a child!

That was one of the nights. Thousands of kilometres away, in the other night, was the small doctor from Prague, the doctor I'd have sunk my teeth in if only I could.

In Prague, too, people couldn't sleep that night. That was the summer when the houses had opened up and released those who had hidden in them with their forbidden thoughts. Daddy shows me the pictures from Prague. His eyes are sad as though they were filled with old embers.

People went wild with joy. Those who were pale, those who were frightened, sang until they were hoarse. People wondered, guessed, sorted out the rumors. They smoked a thousand cigarettes and in some way believed everything that's impossible.

They still believed when they heard the planes that night. The planes that sounded like thunder.

The doctor from Prague wasn't at home. Work at the clinic was developing at a tremendous rate. Everything meshed, each part strengthened the whole. People talked. People experimented. Their energy, released at last, carried them off in a tumultuous mixture of work and politics.

Mummy takes out a few yellowing newspaper cuttings.

The doctor from Prague worked day and night. Far beyond his capacity, beyond the limits of fatigue. Until it was obvious that he had to rest.

When the planes came he was on holiday.

He was with friends somewhere in Yugoslavia. You can imagine what it was like. The doctor sitting at a radio, listening. His friends and his family around him. His friends warn him. They've heard things people have said: Don't go back today! Don't go back!

His bags are packed in the hall. His children have fallen asleep in the armchairs. The doctor turns the knobs. Beyond the atmospheric interference they can hear rasping voices, cries of despair. Soon the radio station must be abandoned. Tanks are rolling along the streets below. People lie down in front of them. The tanks roll on.

The doctor looks up from the radio. His face is grey and his brown eyes look ill. How can anyone ever laugh again? He must go back!

No, the others in the room breathe. It's difficult to breathe. Don't go back! Think of your work, think of what must be done.

But that's precisely the reason. All the documents are in Prague, the case histories, the statistics, everything that's been done to help the children, the crippled children to walk.

But the doctor won't be allowed work again. Not in Prague. Catholics are undesirables.

They talk all through the night and open the window to get in more air they can't breathe. By morning the room is crowded. One of the doctor's assistants, a physical therapist from Prague, is also on holiday with her family.

What are they going to do?

How we believed! How we hoped! Daddy closes the album full of photos. I've taken it out of the cupboard. It's on the desk in front of me. Across the hard cardboard cover I've written: Asa's Journal.

A child was made.

In Prague people dreamed of a new era. In the soft grass by the River Kalix Mummy and Daddy lay and listened to the voices of people who didn't want to migrate, who wanted to live at home.

In those days people loved the future. And the child would be a child of love! The new life would be created here at home and in Prague. The world would be changed.

I was the child. A broken child. I can see them with their romantic smiles. I can hear their blood bubbling like lemonade. They thought they knew how things were going to turn out.

Chapter Two

If I lean out the window the world becomes bigger. I can see the road. I can feel the moist air against my forehead and cheeks. I can sit like the rabbit, with my nose pushed forward.

The days of my beginning! They knew nothing about a doctor from Prague. Not then. Nor about the expeditions they would make into my brain. They'd all been healthy. Daddy came from a healthy family and so did Mummy. They all grew old as anything. Like old branches in a tree. They withered slowly. They'd all been so healthy they never gave as much as a thought to any other possibility. Why should things change?

A rose climbs up along the wall beneath my window. The petals have fallen. They fall softly. If I lean further out I can fall as they do.

§

I'll take things as they happened, one by one. Mummy became pregnant and was sick. She travelled through the south of Stockholm, through the suburbs, to look at a house. The house was for sale. When she saw the roses she made up her mind at once. Daddy came down from Sherwood Forest.

A house! Are we going to own a house?

Why not? Mummy beamed at him.

Good God!

A lot of people own houses.

Not everyone. Not us.

Daddy stood outside the gate. What was left of the gate. Most of it had rotted and fallen to the ground.

You can sit and write in the room facing south.

Daddy climbed reluctantly over the bits of plank that had been the gate. The garden was full of old timber, a rusty bath tub, pipes that had been torn out, the bottom of a bed, and the remains of a gas heater.

Of course it was wonderful!

A red timber house with pear trees that leaned in over the sharply pitched roof. Old windows with glazing bars and small square panes that glittered in the sun.

Outside the kitchen door was a corner with a little veranda. Daddy put his hand on the railing. It broke off and fell to the ground.

It can be repaired. And if you forget about the rubbish . . . It can be repaired. Say that it's marvellous!

Our flat in town is good enough.

But it wasn't. It faced onto a dark courtyard. Spiked fences separated the neighboring courtyards. A small boy had fallen over one of the fences and been pierced by the spikes.

Mummy opens the kitchen door.

Has the house been inspected? Daddy asks, trying to make his voice sound businesslike and technical. Somewhere or other he's heard that houses should be inspected.

He intended this as an objection. But in fact it was his first step of retreat. Like letting a door-to-door salesman put his foot across the threshold. Mummy immediately pulled out a report of which they understood practically nothing. There was a little dampness in the basement but she brushed past that. A flue pipe in the chimney had cracked. But the other flue pipes could probably be used.

And the windows?

They both looked uncertainly at the windows. Would they fall out as soon as they were touched?

Of course we have to repaint them.

Daddy looked down at his hands. He has big hands. He's strong and he can lift people on one arm. He's made for mending leaks, laying pipes, laying floors.

He shivered. What he wanted to do most of all was to sit at his typewriter and think about philosophy and love.

At any rate the roof doesn't leak!

Hmm, Daddy said. He looked thoughtful. It's important that roofs don't leak. One can put up with most things, but not with a roof that leaks. He was silent for a moment. He needed to think. The situation required mature consideration.

But in fact it was all decided. As soon as Mummy saw the roses it was decided. She stood in the middle of the floor, small and round with all her eagerness in her eyes. Wallpaper peeled from the walls all about her. She didn't care. She has the ability to see beyond things like that. The sun poured in through the windows and lit up Mummy's hair. She has red hair with a green tuft at the top.

Daddy began to laugh. He went up to a wall and thumped it and shouted and laughed. Mortar fell off the wall.

You're out of your mind! Let's buy the house! We're both out of our minds!

Mummy threw her arms around Daddy.

They hugged each other and then they did it there amongst the rubbish on the floor. When I was small I thought that was awful. The idea that Mummy and Daddy did it. But I've got used to it.

They lay on the floor and kissed and undressed each other.

Daddy whispered something. It had something to do with the basement. Mummy giggled and pulled down his underpants. He has green underpants with long legs that end down at his knees. He always wears them and they're the ugliest underpants in the world. I think there was a fire once in a warehouse. He must have bought up the whole stock. I can't understand how one can love someone who wears underpants like that.

Are you sure the roof doesn't leak?

Daddy caressed her breasts. She has small breasts with long nipples. When it's cold her nipples stick out like little pegs. They wound themselves around each other and rolled about on the floor. They were going to begin their life now, their real life.

But what about the money? And the dampness in the basement?

Their questions ended up unanswered in the recess where the tiled stove stood. No one was listening anymore. They were breathing fast and calling words that had no meaning.

Anyway. To buy a house you must have money. And houses that are almost collapsing cost a lot of money. Afterwards they lay side by side on the floor for a while. They caressed each other and thought of money. They were comnists at that time. My intelligent sister would say c-o-m-m-u-n-i-s-t-s and smile her prettiest and coolest smile. I'm almost certain they were comnists. The banks would say no. Why should banks lend money to comnists? If the comnists win, they're going to take over the banks.

There were relatives who could help. After all, it wasn't such an awful lot. They got up and dressed with fumbling hands. They were marvellously happy.

§

A little further away the landscape opens towards a park. Everything in the park is round and gentle, the grassy hills roll in under the trees. Deer used to roam around here long ago.

You can smell the water.

They moved into the house and all the smells of autumn stood outside to bid them welcome. Like servants or something, Mummy laughs as she remembers. The smell of water from the lake, the smell of apples and pears, the smell of wet leaves, the autumn that flickered and burned.

In fact they didn't so much move in as swarm in. They swarmed in with their children and their horde of friends who were supposed to help. They've always had children hanging around them. Mummy had two from before and Daddy had one.

The children are big now. Lisa has become as beautiful as a swan. She knows everything. You can ask her things grown-ups don't understand. But in those days she was small and her nose ran. She was bandy-legged and was always screaming. I don't know Patrick. Patrick is a pretty ridiculous name. Now he's gone abroad. He was another one that screamed a lot. He went out stealing mopeds in the evening. The third child, Olle, was with them that day. Otherwise he usually lived with his mother.

What would people think?

Neighbors gathered at the fences and stared. Daddy drove up in the bus he'd borrowed from the theater. There was a picture on the bus. The bus had once been used for carrying biscuits. The name of the biscuit firm was written in pink letters along the sides. The rest was rust and oil that leaked and smoke that slowly settled over the area.

The whole crowd poured out of the bus. Of course the neighbors began to wonder. Mummy, with her red-green hair and shining like a torch, led the way, the children behind her. She had another child in her stomach.

People thought there was something fishy about it. Proper people have a home, a caravan for holidays, and two children at the most. In the old days social workers went around with information to people who had more than two —people who couldn't restrain themselves.

Lisa was ashamed. There are times when I've been ashamed too. I wish I had parents I could explain. I can't explain my parents and I know already that my story isn't going to do it either.

In real stories you know where you have people. And

real authors are like tailors. They cut out characters, make temperaments to measure and sew on virtues the way you sew on pockets. I have to do a jigsaw puzzle with pieces that must be forced into place because they don't fit.

Mummy and Daddy took over the house. They spread their incredible confusion everywhere. And yet. In the middle of it all there was always a sort of line of development, a direction. That's one of the things that can't be explained.

The house smiled and all the scents of autumn bowed.

Mummy sat inside the window and rested her sickness and her pregnancy. What happiness! She heard the children rush upstairs and take over rooms. Daddy directed the Rabble. They toiled away. The garden was cleared of rubbish. Bushes appeared. There were raspberry bushes! Someone found the last raspberry of the season.

Right in the center of the big room was where Mummy's easel would stand. Mummy furnished the room with her eyes. There, against the bright wall, was room for the angled drawing board. She didn't go in for sitting much. But now she had to rest.

Women love moving. They lie in bed in the mornings and read the housing ads. It's an instinct they have. Searching for a nest, recreating the moment when a home comes into existence. It's an instinct women have, Daddy claims. He reads the car ads.

To begin from the beginning! Daddy stood in front of her. He took hold of her shoulder. She was so absent she might have been asleep.

He had bottles and glasses. It was time to celebrate.

No, she didn't want anything to drink.

But she must join in.

They sat on beer crates and used chipboards as a table. The Rabble sang and cheered. Daddy was going to write a play about a big strike. I think they sang the *Marseillaise* that night.

Between the wine bottles and the candles, they could

glimpse the apple trees outside the window. Imagine carrying big cauldrons to the cooker and making apple sauce!

It must have been around then I got my ears and fingers. I lay like a big shrimp in there where it was warm and heard things. They say the fetus likes to hear friendly sounds.

§

There was one sound I didn't hear. That was the whistle of the train. Nobody in the room heard how the train whistled and roared in a railway station in Yugoslavia. The doctor from Prague got on the train with his wife and his children. Helping hands passed in their luggage.

Not that they had much in the way of luggage. Holiday clothes, a few essentials. From now on their life would be an endless holiday. An endless running away. The doctor leaned out through the train window and held his friends' hands. When you travel you want to take something of your friends with you. So you touch them.

Prague had fallen silent. No one came to their aid. No one would ever come to their aid.

The train rolled out of the station with the doctor and his family. Mummy dreamed about apple sauce.

Daddy sat on the edge of the bed. He felt Mummy's stomach carefully.

There's not much to feel. Not at the beginning. He winked at her in the darkness.

What have we done? he said.

Something good. She fell asleep.

§

Mummy had imagined a different home.

She tore down old wallpaper and put her easel where she wanted it. They had almost no furniture. She liked it best that way. Floors are for walking on. You should be able to walk around in rooms and look at them from new angles. Furniture only gets in the way.

Daddy came home and tore down more wallpaper. He looked at the few pieces of furniture she had arranged, a table and a few kitchen chairs. Then he moved them.

When he'd gone, she moved them back.

They didn't fight with each other. Not so much. They moved furniture and felt their way, tested each other's reactions. They were going to live together now. Before they lived from day to day. Now things were going to be done properly.

How is one to put up with being with the same person all the time? Jesus never had to answer that. He was never forced to look for his sandals or ask who forgot to put the cap on the toothpaste tube.

If only they'd been strong and calm and secure!

They stood poised on the most impossible footholds, they climbed far out to look at views and enjoy dreams and fantasies.

But out there they became each other's victims. Mummy dreamed about white rooms and vast, uncluttered surfaces. She dreamed about apple sauce. In the garden the apples had fallen. She didn't have time to do anything with them. She blamed her lack of time. Pears rained down from the big pear tree. They piled up in great drifts across the grass and rotted. It was impossible to walk on the grass anymore. It was like walking in muck. And there was a smell of fermentation from it.

There were piles of things on the floor. Things have to be put somewhere. Then they lay everywhere, even on the stairs. Mummy stepped like a stork between the piles. She didn't see them.

They competed with each other. They competed with strength, but mostly with inferiority. They made themselves as inferior as little children. I think they needed comforting.

Daddy dreamed about something he called an ordinary

life. They were going to become ordinary people. I can see him now as he, too, steps around like a stork. He does it inside himself. He'll never put things in order inside himself. He steps over all the rubbish he has in there and pretends he's someone he can never become.

When he stumbles over something, he starts a row. Mummy sulks.

Mummy arranged a school for Patrick. There was a school nearby. Our school. But Mummy was careful in those days. The headmaster of the school was known. He used to pull the hair of troublesome children. Outside the school he'd arranged a playground divided into squares.

What's wrong with a playground? Daddy said.

That headmaster's out of his mind, Mummy said. He's forbidden the pupils to form student councils. He refuses to print the school register to prevent angry parents ringing each other.

Daddy became unsure. It sounded odd. But on the other hand, maybe it wouldn't do any harm if Patrick had his hair pulled a little now and then.

He didn't say that. You don't say things like that.

We can send Patrick to the Waldorf School, Mummy said.

Daddy made a face. He walked around the room kicking chairs Mummy had moved. A private school!

It's a good school, Mummy said.

It's run by a religious sect, theosophists or astrologists or something.

Anthroposophists, Mummy said.

Grasseaters.

They're not vegetarians. Mummy tried to keep calm.

It's twenty kilometres to that school! I know how Daddy talked that time because he still talks the same way. The kids won't be allowed to look at TV.

What difference does that make?

I want to see the sports news, Daddy said.

We can hide the TV. We can keep it in the wardrobe in the room upstairs.

Just like the Pentacostal Movement! They've forbidden TV as well. That's why they have their TV sets in the wardrobe.

What does the Pentacostal Movement have to do with this?

Am I supposed to sit in the wardrobe and look at the sports news?

That'd be a relief, Mummy said.

The kid is going to an ordinary school.

Don't call him the kid. His name is Patrick.

You know . . . Daddy raised his voice. He raised his voice and his arms up towards a heaven that doesn't exist: You know what sort of people send their kids to that school?

Good people, I'm sure, Mummy said resolutely.

Far from it. People who can't take care of their own children. They imagine their kids are fragile as glass. You can't touch them. Their silly kids can't stand being told off. That's why they scream and become unpleasant. No one can put up with them. So they're sent away.

I think the Waldorf School would be good, Mummy said.

The kids will be marked for life, Daddy said. They're given special treatment. After that they never get off the analyst's couch.

Ordinary people were what they were going to become. Daddy kept repeating that. The kids are going to go to an ordinary school. A local school. And kick ordinary footballs. Go to the school nurse if they hurt themselves. Go home during the break and steal biscuits.

Ordinary biscuits, Mummy said.

Exactly!

Mummy got up. It was becoming more difficult for her to get up. But she hadn't grown fatter. Not that you could see. The tiredness came first, a tiredness that wasn't like any other tiredness she had ever felt.

Daddy made her tired. Does one have to become ordinary? She looked out the window. Daddy had made an effort to dig the apples off the lawn. He was trying to be practical and the effort discouraged him. He'd thrown the shovel amongst the apples and gone in to write a poem about the liberation of the workers instead.

The neighbors had stopped staring. Their first disquiet had calmed down. But Mummy had already been reprimanded. She'd hung out the wash on a Sunday.

Patrick was allowed to begin in a local school. But not the one closest to us. He was sensitive. He couldn't stand having his hair pulled when he stole mopeds. Lisa started at the day nursery.

§

I kicked. It happened when autumn grew cold and grey. Mummy stayed in bed. She crept down under the eiderdown. She had a tray beside her. She put out her hands and picked food and put it in her mouth.

You get so hungry.

It's awful to be pregnant. You feel sick all the time. Not the usual way, but in a new way. Nauseous! So you eat to stop it. Everything you eat is to press down the nausea. Mummy ate oranges. The thought of sweet, juicy oranges made her almost sick with longing.

She loves to lie under her eiderdown. Now she lay there and decided to think happy thoughts. She didn't think about the boiler that had broken down. Or about the electric wiring that had burnt up. Daddy had run a cable directly from the basement so that they could cook.

She ate, shovelling food into her mouth with one hand. She thought of how marvellous it is to eat. And of Daddy coming with the tray in the morning. He was always attentive to her in one way or another.

She thought of how he took Lisa to the day nursery. He

was careful about that sort of thing as well. Share and share alike.

If only she didn't have to get out of bed her happiness would be complete. It was at precisely that moment, when she lay back on the pillow, that she felt the kick. At first you don't really know what it is. It might be something else, like when your stomach rumbles, but further down. You should preferably be quite still and it's best if there's no noise.

She felt the kick. Such a light kick! As though a butterfly struck you with his wing. Once and, after a little while, once again.

She turned round and got up on all fours amongst the crumbs and orange peel in the bed. She took a deep breath and pushed her foot out into the coldness of the room.

At the beginning you stand naked in front of the mirror. Nothing, or almost nothing, can be seen. You just have a memory of the light stroke of the butterfly's wing. She pushed out her stomach. Now it could be seen clearly.

That's the way women stand. Imagine if you could collect them all in a big room just when they're standing naked in front of their mirrors and pushing out their stomachs and listening! The happy ones together with the panic-stricken.

Being pregnant, Mummy says, it's not awful at all.

§

They painted the big room. Almost everything was painted, the wainscot, the skirting, the old piping. They used thick, soft rollers to paint with and everything became white.

They painted at night. The days were for rushing out into the world. The world out there! Maybe you have the idea Mummy lay all day long amongst the breadcrumbs in her bed. Maybe it sounds like that. But that wasn't the way it was. She used her morning lie-ins to listen inwards.

In reality they were endlessly active. They ran through what was out there. They held onto their dreams the way you hold onto flags that flutter in the wind. They shook them the way people shake out bedclothes. The more impossible something seemed, the more eager they became.

In some way this too is part of my story. What they were like, what everything was like out there, outside the stomach where I lay, outside the white walls they painted.

Mummy was mixed up in Daddy's theater. But mostly she made clothes. She designed clothes that were pretty and soft. Sort of political clothes. Clothes people would wear when the revolution came. The clothes were called The Wardrobe of Celestial Peace. Something Chinese.

Daddy didn't wear them. He tried once. That was just after they'd fallen in love with each other. He bought a green suit from Mummy. It looked mad, he says. The suit didn't fit his long, bony body. Mummy's political clothes were made for small, slim people. But he wore the suit out of love for her.

One evening his trousers split. They divided in two. They split from the fly all the way 'round up to the belt at the back. Daddy was standing on Stureplan, one of the busiest streets of Stockholm. The taxis refused to pick him up.

When he got home Mummy took out a measuring tape and measured him. From then on she designed the big suits to his measurements. So a lot of people walked around dressed in Celestial clothes that were tailored to fit Daddy.

Everyone except Daddy.

Mummy held political meetings. When Daddy was out travelling, people came home to us and drank tea. They read little red books that had been written by the fat Chinaman. I call them Mummy's politicals.

They were an odd lot, Daddy says.

Not in the least, Mummy says.

A lot of them were odd. They drank tea. They didn't say

hello when I walked into the room. They looked at me peculiarly. They didn't shake hands.

You're exaggerating, Mummy says.

Her nose is fairly small and it seems to become smaller and sharper when she grows angry. Apart from that, you can't see when she's angry. Apart from that, her anger is turned inwards. But I can see it from her nose. Some of them might have been odd. But they weren't all odd.

The dreams weren't odd either, she says. Far away. . . . She sits beside her window and listens to the branches of the pear tree rustle against the roof. There was a country far away. No, not Prague with the gloomy clouds. Another country. The story she tells is like a saga about shepherd lads and lasses who hide down the well and hear a giant tramp about above them. You can imagine this country when you look past her and out through the window. People run around, men and women dressed in black run around, you hear the giant's steps, you hear the shepherd lad blow his horn. He climbs up on the giant's foot. The freedom fighters rush forward, towns are stormed, foreigners are put to flight, the impossible happens. For real? Was it for real? She smiles. She's lost in distant memories.

Some went crazy, Daddy says.

Some who?

Of us. Of them. He talks about the man who thought he was a cock. Early one Sunday morning they were awakened by a noise on the staircase. It was when they lived in town. It sounded like cackling.

They opened the door and out there stood one of Mummy's politicals. He was naked. He'd glued Easter feathers all over his body. They invited him in and tried to talk to him. But his only response was to cluck and crow. Then he opened a window and jumped out into the courtyard. He disappeared and never came back.

Everyone laughs when Daddy tells this story. Everyone except Mummy.

Or the man with the bag. Late one evening someone rang

at the door. There was a man out there in the dark talking. He'd pulled a bag over his head. He said he was being persecuted by American spies. Mummy invited him in. They sat in the kitchen and drank tea and the man kept the bag over his head all the time. He said they sprayed poisonous gas into his home. He wanted Daddy to write something. The American spies sprayed poisonous gas in through cracks in the roof and walls.

Everyone laughs again. Mummy gets up and leaves the room. She doesn't look at Daddy. She's not feeling well.

They tell their stories. As though they lived on stories and fantasies. But they don't seem to be in agreement. Not anymore. I lie in Mummy's stomach and she feels the beat of the butterfly's wings. Outside is the white room and outside the room all sorts of things are happening. I think they're part of my story.

I talk about things I don't understand. Daddy was in Skövde several times that autumn. When he wasn't writing his play about the big strike, he travelled to Skövde with his typewriter. That's one event that's in the album with the cuttings. Skövde lay in Sherwood Forest and he was going to help liberate a few charwomen there.

They were working in a hotel and they suffered from backache. They were thinking of going on strike. Daddy wrote in the newspaper and the strike broke out. The whole thing was a great scandal. A woman who was a minister in the Labor Government was staying at the hotel when the strike broke out. Her bed wasn't made that morning.

There was a court case. Daddy's article was used in the court as evidence. There's a big picture of the charwomen above the article in the album with the cuttings. The minister was very upset. A lot of people were appalled. Charwomen going on strike! Whatever next! Who's going to do the cleaning if charwomen go on strike? The minister's bed wasn't made for several days. The charwomen's action had to be condemned. As a warning to others.

Daddy's eyes light up. He has fantasies of his own he lives on. But then suddenly he begins to swear. Damn, he says. Bloody hell. The light in his eyes goes out.

I was kicking more now. *That's* part of my story. Like the house and Aunt Tilly.

§

The doctor from Prague listened to the thump of the rails. Yellow lamps shot flashes of light into the carriage as the train rushed through nameless villages and towns. The bells howled at the level crossings and the world cried. The children slept huddled up like fetuses on the seats. Imagine sleeping like them! Wretched Europe where no one can sleep anymore. Where people were afraid of ghosts at night and hoped they wouldn't see the new day with all its disappointments.

Prague was shut down. The city had been shut down and now it lay there like a mussel in its hard shell of evil. Everything abandoned! Saying those words is one thing, understanding them is another. An exile is never understood by those who have a home and a history to return to.

The doctor and his wife sat opposite each other on the seats by the window. They closed their eyes and tried to fool each other into believing that they were asleep. They tried, but they didn't succeed.

You should sleep now.

Yes, I should.

You're skeptical?

Who isn't skeptical?

She reached out her hand and put it on his knee. An exile's hand, she thought.

Everything abandoned!

She looked around the carriage. Her youngest child lay with its hand under its cheek. She looked at her husband with his gentle eyes. Not everything. Not what was most important.

The doctor smiled at his wife. The pale smile of the exile. His lips moved but his words were drowned in the clatter from the railway station. We're not travelling alone.

They comforted each other as they had comforted each other in the last few days. The doctor moved over and sat beside her. They repeated words, old words they had already pushed back and forth between them. They had friends in Cologne. They'd settle down there.

The doctor huddled up and shivered. He was sacrificing his family for his own wild ambition. He was cutting off their roots and dragging them out in a flight that had no end.

They'd never have let you work at home, she said.

There are other kinds of work.

Not for you. She sounded calm, sensible. But deep in the shadows she cried for the second time these last few days. She had cried the first time when the radio fell silent. She said, you are the servant of the Lord. So are we.

They had their love, their understanding. They were travelling on a secret mission. They were smuggling love and understanding across the borders like contraband goods.

The world comes apart. What is dear to you lies on a street bleeding. I think of Mummy and Daddy and the doctor and how they travelled through the world in the same carriage. A dream train rolls through the world on rails of fantastic hopes.

The world is chaos and the house is chaos. The electric wiring has burnt up. There aren't enough cupboards and wardrobes. There's nowhere to put your things, nowhere you can be.

And yet! Precisely at that moment when everything seems to be torn apart. Precisely then! There was that strange faith that would make me scream so that blood ran from my mouth, so that my eyes were turned inside out.

Chapter Three

They'd had their period of gingerly feeling their way forward. Now it was over.

Daddy kicked at the piles of clothes Mummy had placed on the stairs. He stormed through the rooms and talked about the proper life that he'd just begun. They were going to live like civilized beings. They were going to clean up and wake early in the morning. They were going to do the dishes straight after dinner and educate Patrick.

The autumn was unspeakably cold. No one could remember such an ice-cold autumn.

Daddy ran up the stairs with long strides. After him came Mummy on her short legs.

You must tidy up after you! Daddy told her what was what. The day of judgment had arrived.

Don't sound so grumpy, Mummy called from behind his back.

I'm not grumpy!

You're sulky and you're behaving badly.

Daddy stopped in his tracks. He had a pain in his head. It felt like it was bursting. He'd intended to rush up to Patrick to educate him. Now he turned around to educate Mummy instead.

You must tidy up!

Stop shouting at me!

Daddy bent down and picked up a pile of clothes from the floor and threw them over the balustrade.

What are you doing?

Those clothes shouldn't be lying here!

Are they better lying at the bottom of the stairs?

Mummy's red hair glowed angrily. She said Daddy should mend the electric wiring instead of kicking up a fuss.

Daddy can look awful. His face becomes like old ice.

Get rid of the apples in the garden, Mummy went on. She turned his attack against him. Put in new wiring, mend the boiler.

Daddy went slowly down the stairs and into the big room, the white room. The layer of ice around him grew as thick as armor. Who can educate women? They can no more be educated than cats can. That's the sort of thing he says when he thinks only Mummy can hear him.

You must once have had a tidying-up trauma, he said. Some time in your childhood you suffered a trauma. You've been injured, it's damaged your brain. You don't see what it looks like.

Can't we be pleasant to each other? Mummy said. Do you have to go on complaining?

I want to be able to walk around in this place.

There's nothing stopping you from walking around, Mummy said.

The place should be kept clean. He pointed at the slut's wool in the corners. Someone had reported Mummy to the social welfare people. A lady had been home to baby-sit with Lisa when Lisa had a cold. The lady reported Mummy. She said it was dirty in our house. The lady ran her fingers along the tops of mouldings and cupboards.

Clean up yourself, Mummy said.

Am I supposed to go around cleaning up your rubbish? I'm supposed to put in the new wiring.

But you're not doing it, Mummy said.

They tormented each other. They searched for faults that couldn't be remedied. They lay in wait for each other.

We're freezing to death, Mummy said.

I should hope so, Daddy told her.

What do you want? What are you really after? Mummy

tried to coax him. That's one of the differences between them. He waits behind his ice, he waits for her to begin to coax. Then he puts up resistance.

An ordinary proper life. He talked about the ordinary proper life he dreamed of. He sat on the very edge of a chair.

You're becoming neurotic about ordinariness, Mummy said.

He wanted curtains. They'd painted the big room white. He didn't like it. He preferred wallpaper with flowers or fabric on the walls.

Mummy shivered.

He wanted a nice home. He wanted it to be snug and cozy.

Mummy looked as if she were face to face with a hijacker.

I agreed to it being painted white, Daddy said. He thought she had good taste. Mummy'd attended art school. She'd been trained to have good taste. That was why she was allowed to decide.

It's that damned architect, Daddy said. She'd been married to an architect. It was the architect who'd ruined her.

She didn't answer.

Architects are the worst of all. They design rooms you can't even be in. In their world you're supposed to look at rooms, not be in them. And when it comes to chairs! Architects make chairs you can't sit on.

We don't need curtains, Mummy said. We have flowers.

Daddy laughed a bitter, cutting laugh. He walked up to the windows and poked at Mummy's plants. They're dead, he said.

I don't believe that, Mummy said.

Dead as a doornail. As though they'd never been alive.

Daddy poked at the yellowing remnants of leaves and stems. Mummy winced. It was as though he had poked inside her. Where she really lived, the life that only existed in her head. He opened the window and began to throw out the pots.

What are you doing? The words came in a whisper. You could hear the pots crash outside.

Action was what remained. Action was the means he would use to put life in order. The life neither of them controlled.

He rushed up to the chairs, the loathsome chairs the architect had thought up to torment his fellow human beings. Every time you sat down on them a bit of your backbone was ground away. The architect had won a prize for the chairs.

Daddy struck one of the chairs against the floor and broke a leg. Then he broke the other legs, one by one.

Things are quiet in the area where we live. People say it's one of the quietest districts around. The children are all clean and tidy. On Sundays their fathers repair the family cars and the mothers drink coffee. No one strolling through the area can guess what it's really like, what it's like to break chairs and chase each other up and down the staircase.

Adults catalogue each other's weaknesses. They make lists that are longer than lists of what one would like for Christmas. They classify each other's characteristics. They build a chamber of horrors around themselves. They put monster mummies and monster daddies with cracked eyes and sharp teeth on long rows of shelves.

They do this by their own free choice. They live their lives the way they want to live them. Sometimes they emerge from the chamber of horrors, the chamber they create for themselves in their imagination, and say that they love each other. I don't understand it. I'll never understand it.

Daddy threw the rest of the chairs out the window. He pulled the table to one side and pointed at the wall where Mummy's easel stood. She hadn't had time to use it. But she felt the same sensual pleasure every time she saw it.

Don't touch the easel, she shouted. It was a cry of distress. If you do . . .

If I do?

She didn't know. She could always run away from home, he suggested. A lot of women run away. You hear their descriptions on the radio.

No wonder, Mummy said. Their husbands are unbearable.

Or she could join the Association for the Preservation of Dirt in the Home, he said.

He pointed to where the easel stood. But he didn't touch it. Here was where they should have a TV. A color TV.

And in front of the TV, big soft armchairs. And a sofa, a soft chubby sofa you can sink down into and lie on.

While I clean up! Mummy's nose was sharper than ever and her voice was as poisonous as the color of the green tuft in her hair.

At that very moment the world burst into our house. There was a knock at the door and Mummy's politicals were there with their little red books. They'd come to discuss the peoples' struggle, the world's struggle. They stood in the big room and looked at what was left of the chairs Daddy hadn't yet had time to throw out the window.

Don't mind all that, Mummy said. He's just breaking up the house.

That was her revenge. Daddy felt it like a cramp in his chest. Mummy usually gets her revenge by telling other people what he does.

It doesn't matter, one of the politicals said.

What is it that doesn't matter? Daddy asked threateningly.

We can sit on the floor.

They sat on the floor. Mummy went out to the kitchen and made tea. Daddy went down to the basement. Emotions raged around the cramp in his chest. All he had done was try to be normal. Someone must be normal when everyone else is abnormal. One must learn to deal with life.

But Mummy didn't want to. Daddy was bourgeois, she used to say.

He fled down into the basement and talked to himself. He usually talks to himself when he's been offended. Bourgeois! The word came out with a squeak. It must mean something terrible.

Is it bourgeois to clean up? Everyone has to clean up. It's only the upper classes who don't need to clean up. They have servants. He talked to the basement walls and got answers. He wanted revenge. He wanted to find something, a killing blow. Flowers need to be watered, bread should be buttered properly, people should eat up their food. That was it. People shouldn't poke at their food.

He almost became excited. He was working up a new monster mummy on the shelf in the basement, one who pokes at her food. He was going to show her what she was like. He decided to buy black pudding.

Mummy hates black pudding. He thought he'd make a dinner with black pudding, arrange a day of judgment. It was time to show Mummy what she was really like. And black pudding was the thing to do it with. To show her how finicky, spoiled, and stuck-up she was.

Feeling good again because of his plan, he regarded the basement. An old oil-fired boiler stood in one corner, leaking. He didn't dare put on the boiler. But it would have to be put on sooner or later. The autumn was terribly cold and the cold and moisture crept over the floors and into their very hearts.

Now he was going to show them! Now he was going to be a responsible father, a father who kept his family warm. He searched through a cupboard and found a pair of pliers. He weighed the pliers in his hand. They'd do fine.

He knew nothing about pliers. Or about tools. He hadn't the faintest idea about things like that. He put the pliers around the leaking coupling and began to pull it tight.

With a crunching sound, the coupling thread gave way. A jet of water shot out over the basement. He threw himself on top of the pipe and put his palm against the opening. He began to sweat. He stood quite still for a long time with his hand against the pipe. The sweat poured down his brow and he groaned. A naked bulb spread its gloomy light over the basement. Hell doesn't exist, he thought, but if it did this is what it would look like.

He knew he'd have to call for help. But he put off calling to the people who were upstairs as long as possible. He let go of the pipe and while the water gushed out he ran around under the house. There must be a main valve somewhere. Every house has a main valve. When he finally found it, he discovered it had rusted solid.

They heard his shouts and came down. It would have been better if he'd stayed underground forever. But Mummy didn't say a word of what he'd expected her to say. She has a generous heart. She's not like him. He sat huddled up amongst the pipes like a big, wet lizard while she took care of him and mothered him.

She needed his weakness. That's the way it was. She needed him just as he was at that moment.

Her political friends stood around in a ring. They knew nothing about pipes. The fat Chinaman wrote nothing about pipes in his red books. Maybe, one of her politicals suggested, they could take a cork and use it to plug the hole.

Luckily, there are plumbers. Somewhere there's always a plumber for people like that, a plumber on night duty. While Daddy was waiting for the plumber, Mummy ran up and down the stairs. She fed him chocolate balls covered with dried coconut. Patrick had made them. She brought him wine. He ate the chocolate balls and drank the red wine. They relieved some of his suffering.

Mummy made him happy.

The water rose around his feet. Just now he was beaten. But he'd make a comeback. He thought of Mummy. They'd met when the students had occupied a building, the student union building.

They become embarrassed when they talk about how they met. Not just embarrassed. They giggle as though they had secrets to hide.

The students were angry. The ones who were most angry ran to the Chinese Embassy and tore down the curtains. Only the bourgeoisie have curtains, the students shouted.

Perhaps that's where Mummy got her dislike of curtains. He had water in his shoes and he heard how it squished when he moved his feet.

Mummy had looked Chinese. She'd put lots of black make-up over her eyes. She had slanted eyes. That was the first thing you noticed. She looked exotic. Mongolian folds, she called it. An old doctor had said she had Mongolian folds in the corner of her eyes. And she had two small dimples where her back ends above her behind. Like the Mongolians, the doctor said.

She'd shown him the dimples the very first evening he got at her. They were like the dimples people get when they laugh. She had dimples like that in her behind.

Mummy had black eyes and false eyelashes. She had a small black skirt. In those days skirts ended well above the knees. She fluttered her long eyelashes and seduced him.

After a while, Mummy washed her face. She took off the false eyelashes. Her political friends didn't like make-up. Nor did they approve of drinking wine. So Mummy had to drink wine in secret. When her politicals had finished their tea and gone home to bed, Daddy and Mummy sneaked out their bottles. Sometimes I think everything they did was underhanded. That's why they giggle and get stars in their eyes when they remember.

When the plumber had mended the boiler they went up to the bedroom. There they made love. They're crazy about making love. They're so childish. They fight a whole day and then they make love with each other.

Exhausted, they sank down together on the bed. They became a single being wailing words of love.

I know, I've heard how they sound. They wailed and

Mummy cried. They had that in common, they had that to give each other.

And me, they had me. Daddy knelt in the bed. He pulled the blanket over him like a tent. He listened. He'd heard somewhere that you should listen with a tube. So he listened through an empty toilet paper roll. He put it against Mummy's stomach and listened.

In there he heard a pulse. He heard a heart.

Oh! he said almost soundlessly.

He put on the light and placed his watch in front of him in the bed. He took Mummy's wrist and counted her pulse beats. Then he listened again to her stomach through the roll. He counted the weak, almost inaudible beats.

I can hear the child's heart. One hundred thirty-seven beats a minute.

They laughed. He switched off the light. Their laughter was soft like pigeons cooing. Happily they bid this new life welcome. They didn't know.

Would they have laughed if they had known? There are parents who have their child aborted when they suspect there's something wrong with it.

§

The weather grew colder. Daddy's shelf of monsters grew bigger. He pottered about on his shelf and changed Mummy. Her eyes weren't exotic. They were small and piercing. On one shelf he kept one of her many heads, a head like a pig's with small, listless eyes. On another shelf he had an old lizard, a green prehistoric lizard with short legs and a mouth full of short teeth. This shelf of monsters was his very own. Mummy suspected that it existed, but she wasn't allowed to see it, not even when they fought.

She tended her white room. And her disorder. There's no need to clean up nonstop. One should concentrate on what's important in life.

I know how she thinks. She gathers together her children

and shares her time with them. This happens at the dinner table. There's a moment which is ours. A moment that requires peace and tranquility. Children need that. You don't jump up and start washing the dishes when you sense a black shadow above a child's head. A lot of mothers wash up to avoid things like that. They escape into the washing up when they sense shadows. Mothers like that get children who tell lies.

Mummy's children never lie to her. No matter what they do, even the very worst things, they tell her about them. She listens and touches their hearts. She's like a burglar. When no one is looking she sneaks around and picks locks. She opens up the children and looks into them.

Daddy said it was time to clear the table.

Let's sit a while longer, Mummy answered.

Patrick must help.

Yes, yes, Mummy said.

They were going to become like normal children. Children should set the table and wash up. They should do their lessons and go to bed at half-past eight.

Mummy got up. She left the kitchen, she left the dirty dishes and what was left of the food and sat at the window in the big room. She'd moved a few chairs in there.

Normal upbringing, Daddy said from the kitchen.

Mummy had Patrick and Lisa with her beside the window. You shouldn't order children to do things. That's what she thought. You shouldn't govern and manage them. Not so much anyway.

One should concentrate on what's important in life.

Daddy had recovered after his defeat in the basement. The water had ebbed away. It disappeared slowly, which indicated some sort of block in the drain. Now it had all gone.

Other disasters were on their way. And more water. The house whimpered. It was neither autumn nor winter. It was nothing and it struck again and again. It was the wind that howled and the branches that beat against the metal roof. It was water, rivers of ice-cold water that cascaded down the windows. There was something wrong. There was something wrong with the gutters.

This something, there was always this dark something.

The boiler gasped and hissed as though it were ill. If you put your hand against the radiators you could feel the heat, a weak heat like the flicker of life in a dying breath. It was almost impossible to stay indoors. Mummy held onto the window sill. She was already abnormally big. She had difficulty breathing, she was too tired to breathe.

Must one change? A husband comes storming into one's life, rumbling and roaring like the autumn winds outside the windows. Why can't one live the way one is? Husbands rumble and one must close one's ears to keep the noise out. One can decide to ignore it. Husbands carry their burden of desolate silence and when things become too silent, they rumble.

She was determined not to give way. Men aren't prepared for the obstinacy women can show. She sat on a mountain of tough, almost indestructible obstinacy. When the storm has died down, you can pick stones on the beach. They lie there in the same way they've always done. The women emerge and everything is just as it has always been.

Daddy left the kitchen with the potato peels and the pork chops that hadn't been finished. He'd tried to teach Patrick to eat the entire chop, but it was impossible. Somewhere in the meat there was always an invisible strip of fat, disgusting fat.

He went down to the basement and puttered about with the monsters on his shelf. He tried to think proper thoughts. His big play about the strike was half finished. It was about a factory and the workers had already begun to discuss it in groups. The New Life! That was a fine name for the play.

He tried to think thoughts like this while the piles of potato peel grew on the kitchen table. They multiplied, filled the kitchen, and slid down the basement steps. The damp concrete walls and the wheezing of the boiler beneath the naked bulb made him think of torture.

How should one organize the new life?

Be comrades. Men and women should also be comrades. Daddy really thought this at the time.

Comrades! He tried out the word on them up there. There was no response.

He's so sensitive, Mummy said. You have to be careful with him.

We must all give a hand, Daddy called.

It's a pity about him, Mummy said. It's his nerves. They're so close to the surface. She could afford to talk like that. She felt like a winner.

They were nearly always quarrelling. But they didn't fight. Not then.

§

It was Aunt Tilly who arrived with the new life. She stood on the steps wearing a fluttering raincoat and with the first of the snow on the kerchief around her head.

Aunt Tilly, how nice! Mummy made an effort to say it but she sounded as false as an actor on the radio.

Here I am, Aunt Tilly said and put one foot across the threshold as though afraid Mummy might close the door.

What a surprise! Daddy threw his arms around Aunt Tilly and pulled her into the hall.

Aunt Tilly is small and thin. She's always carrying lots of paper bags. This time she had more bags than usual and she took them with her into the hall.

What awful weather! She shook herself like a big black bird. It wasn't easy finding you.

But you managed it in the end, Mummy said.

You might have told me, Aunt Tilly said sharply.

Mummy and Daddy looked ashamed. They'd abandoned Aunt Tilly. They'd decided to abandon her for a while. Aunt Tilly let the contents of her bag flow out over the floor. She'd been to a bazaar. The church had had a bazaar in Högalid. They were selling things for the mission. The Negroes were to be Christianized and Aunt Tilly bought things that might be useful.

Aunt Tilly bent down, showing how agile she is for her age. She had plates, checkered plates, cutlery, a coffee pot, vegetable grinders, several of them, and salt cellars. She also had a whole bag with unidentified objects.

It's far too much, Daddy said.

Mummy stiffened from top to toe. She's particular about things. Simple things, white things. She almost gets tears in her eyes, she says there's something about proportions and lines. Now she tried to control her expression while Aunt Tilly showed the presents.

How kind, Mummy said.

Aunt Tilly opened the leather bag she had tied around her stomach. She always has her leather bag tied around her stomach. She says she does it in case there are robbers.

The children were allowed to come near and look into the bag. Aunt Tilly usually has sweets in her bag. She has other things as well, bracelets, bits of glass, small change.

The children stood with their bags of sweets and said thank you. You never know what sort of sweets she has or where she got hold of them. Aunt Tilly's sweets aren't like ordinary sweets. Daddy claims she buys surplus sweets and that she haggles over the price. During the war she bought a load of sweets that had been damaged by seawater. A ship loaded with sweets had been torpedoed. Aunt Tilly was on the spot at once and bought up the whole cargo.

Aunt Tilly hung up her raincoat and unlaced her wet boots. Imagine! Mummy and Daddy were houseowners!

We're so happy, Mummy said. She stood where she was and stared at Aunt Tilly's pile on the floor while Daddy showed Aunt Tilly around the house. Mummy suspected that the day had come, the day she had been fearing.

What a state this place is in! Aunt Tilly said. She stood in the middle of the big room and looked around.

We were just going to clean up, Daddy said. We didn't know you were coming. Let's have coffee.

We must tidy here first, Aunt Tilly said and began to pick things up from the floor at once.

No! Mummy ran in and took hold with both hands of the things Aunt Tilly had picked up. I'll tidy up here. You just sit down and rest.

Aunt Tilly has never rested in her life. She doesn't know what you do when you rest. Mummy pulled at the things but Aunt Tilly was strong. They wrestled silently. Aunt Tilly won.

Anyway, there's nowhere to sit here, she said. There's no furniture.

We haven't had time, Daddy said. He's loyal. It would never occur to him to expose Mummy to the public gaze. He went up to Mummy and hugged her the way you do with people who have suffered unexpected grief. But he didn't seem worried, more in good spirits.

We must see about furniture, Aunt Tilly said.

We'll manage that ourselves, Mummy said. Anyway we don't want much furniture. We like it the way it is.

I'll help you, Aunt Tilly said. She's hard of hearing. She doesn't hear what people say. Sometimes. With her arms full of clothes and other things she'd picked from the floor she climbed the stairs.

Mummy looked after her. What guilt! What shame! Woe to the woman who fails to lavish care on her home! Try to break free, fight your way through invisible barriers, it's all in vain. Sooner or later Aunt Tilly enters your life. Aunt Tilly always wants to help, Mummy said. Aunt Tilly is like those special offers where you fill in the coupon and don't discover until later that you've committed yourself to paying off installments for the rest of your life.

Aunt Tilly is an expert on bad consciences. So Mummy claims. Aunt Tilly creates guilt. That way she improves her own conscience. She clings to the trunks of the big, healthy trees and sucks life from them.

Take it easy, Daddy said.

We don't want her here.

I can't throw her out.

You can ask her to go, Mummy said. Make up some excuse.

No one can get Aunt Tilly to go if she's decided to stay, Daddy said.

You can.

Not even I can.

You don't want to?

Aunt Tilly has her good points, Daddy said. He also had a debt to pay. Aunt Tilly took care of him when he was small when my grandmother and grandfather died and Daddy was left alone.

They both heard how Aunt Tilly rummaged around in the bedroom.

What's she doing up there? Try to get her out of here!

No, we must show some consideration.

To whom?

One doesn't throw out one's childhood. Aunt Tilly was Daddy's childhood. One just has to put up with one's childhood. Everyone must.

Doesn't she have any sensitivity at all? Mummy said.

I don't think so.

Aunt Tilly appeared on the landing. She informed them that she'd taken the opportunity to tidy up the bedroom a little.

There's no need to, Daddy said.

What a state this place is in, Aunt Tilly said.

Mummy's first impulse was to run away. She wanted to run straight out into the slushy snow. But you can't do things like that.

One might be tempted to think that Aunt Tilly is unique, Daddy says, but she's not. If she'd lived in the seventeenth century she'd have pulled a cart across the battle fields. Nowadays women like that don't use carts. They use public transport and they carry paper bags.

I know what we'll do, Aunt Tilly said.

They drank coffee. There was nothing in the kitchen, they had nothing to offer. But Aunt Tilly had thought of that as well. She had a green marzipan cake in the last paper bag that hadn't yet been opened.

It's a little dry, Aunt Tilly said. She'd come across an old cake. They were selling off old cakes in a cake shop on Hornsgatan. Aunt Tilly'd got the cake at half price.

They drank coffee and the children ate up the cake. Children love Aunt Tilly for her cakes and her bags with odd, unusual things. Children are a little afraid of her as well but marzipan is marzipan.

There's nothing wrong with the cake, Aunt Tilly said. It doesn't smell.

Lisa's nose was running as usual. Daddy thought it was because of the day nursery. All the children at day nurseries have running noses.

You must wear warm clothes, Aunt Tilly told Lisa. You must have socks and a warm cardigan.

She'll be all right, Mummy said.

It's so cold here, Aunt Tilly said. The only cure is heat.

I don't think so, Mummy said. A little cold doesn't do any harm. It makes you healthy and tough.

I don't think she looks healthy, Aunt Tilly said. Her nose is running. Aunt Tilly got up, fetched her cardigan and draped it over Lisa's shoulders. Mummy dropped her spoon. She'd tried to taste the cake but couldn't.

What a pleasant evening, Daddy said.

Aunt Tilly beamed contentedly. Now the house was going to be furnished.

§

I think Daddy conspired with Aunt Tilly. He took her on for the job. Mummy thinks so too but she has no proof.

Daddy sometimes says awful things to Aunt Tilly. He's not afraid of saying awful things to her. She rings him up when he's at work. He's sitting at an important meeting. No one is allowed to disturb him. No calls get through.

But Aunt Tilly gets through one way or another. She creeps like a fox terrier along the telephone lines and scents him out. She rings and says she's at Nytorget. Or maybe it's Odengatan. She's standing there and she's just found a refrigerator. A cheap refrigerator.

I don't have time, Daddy says.

You must come with the car, Aunt Tilly says. I can't stand here with the refrigerator all day long.

No, Daddy says.

You need a refrigerator, Aunt Tilly says.

Go to hell, Daddy shouts and slams down the receiver.

Aunt Tilly cries. Daddy's ungrateful. But in the end it doesn't matter. Daddy can say almost anything to her and she still forgives him.

This was the season of darkness, the darkest of the dark. The lights had to be on all day. Daddy shouted at Aunt Tilly and when he wasn't shouting at her he held secret discussions with her.

He'd abandoned his plan with the black pudding. He didn't need to show how Mummy picked at her food. He had Aunt Tilly. She became his will and his eyes in the dark when she travelled by bus through town wearing her kerchief and carrying her bags.

They furnished the house. They furnished my life.

Mummy saw it happen. With blazing eyes she stood in the doorway and tried to stop them from carrying in the big sofa.

A sofa's useful, Daddy said.

Not that sofa, she said.

It's soft and comfortable, Daddy said. At least you can try it.

Mummy wanted to stand in the way but gave up. The children threw themselves jubilantly onto the sofa. It was marvelous! Patrick had been teased because he lived in a funny home without furniture and curtains. There were posters with the fat Chinaman on the walls. At school Patrick was called the Chinaman.

Now there was a big, plump sofa on the floor. You could swing and sway and jump on it. Now Patrick could bring other children home. Now they were becoming like ordinary people.

Mummy laughed sometimes. But even when she was laughing tears could appear.

Take care of your stomach, Daddy said. Take it up and put it to bed. It needs to rest.

Mummy held her stomach with both hands. It was enormous. How could her stomach be so big? She left the room. But she didn't go to bed. She almost never does what Daddy suggests. It's an instinct. She sat in the kitchen and smoked.

Aunt Tilly's piercing eyes penetrated the city's darkness. The furniture that was now arriving was the result of her searches. She was a child of the city. She was proud of being a child of the city. She knew how to get hold of furniture.

Someone died. It might be someone in the house she lived in on the south side of the city. But she found out about others who died as well. People are always dying. And when they do Aunt Tilly is there.

The deceased's estate? Mummy wondered.

No, not quite. You have to be there before it actually becomes an estate. You make enquiries amongst the relatives. Might it be possible to . . . a cupboard maybe or the sofa, the big sofa.

You have to be there before it becomes an estate with official appraisers and relatives who get involved in disputes. You have a couple of hundred dollars with you and buy what you want quickly. Two hundred dollars cash and no need for a receipt. Mummy didn't like it.

That's the way Aunt Tilly is, Daddy said.

Do we have to? Mummy asked, but she was really thinking of something else. Her stomach absorbed all her concentration.

Aunt Tilly isn't wicked, Daddy said.

That may be, Mummy said. But what is she?

A container lady. Daddy knew Aunt Tilly. He could always find just the right thing to compare her with. The world is divided into people who throw things away in containers and those who take things out of the same containers.

When the attics were cleared out in the house where Aunt Tilly lives all the tenants put the things they wanted to throw away down in the courtyard. They all did it, except Aunt Tilly. She rented two new storage areas in the attic and carried what everyone else had thrown away back up again. She carried almost all of it up.

That's what Aunt Tilly's like.

It's something to do with her background. Her background was so poor. Aunt Tilly saves anything that might be useful. She has complete sets of kitchen equipment, children's beds, and all sorts of fittings and furnishings stored in the attic.

The day may well come, she says.

Now the day had come and our house was being furnished. It was all carried in from the darkness outside. It wasn't rubbish, it was almost never rubbish. The sofa looked awful but it was terrific for bouncing up and down on. Then the secretaire came. It has secret compartments and it's antique.

You have to admit that it's a fine piece of furniture, Daddy said.

Mummy heard them carry the things in while she sat in the kitchen with her dreams about a house that refused to become the sort of house she had wanted.

§

That was the way Aunt Tilly created our home and that was the way God created the world. The night has moved on a bit while I've been riffling through their memories. But everything is still the same as it was when I began my story: The rabbit's eyes and the faint sounds from the motorway. There's nothing to hear, no cries and no laughs.

God couldn't afford to buy new things either when He created the world. He should have waited until He could afford it. He could have gone to a place where they sold quality goods. Even cut-price furniture stores have nice things. But He got hold of a few leftovers and He dug the rest out of containers. Why didn't He take more time about it?

Such a lot of things went wrong. And yet He let the child be born.

Chapter Four

It's not going to be easy.

The doctor from Prague perceived the slight shift in tone. He couldn't avoid hearing it. His friends weren't sure, not as sure as they had been. They'd helped him. A lot of help was needed after the long journey. They said how sorry they were and they arranged things for his family.

But his work, that wasn't so certain anymore.

The doctor looked up at the soot-dark sky above Cologne. There was no avoiding the doubts his friends felt. But he reacted as though he didn't notice. Tawny clouds, soot, and factory stacks hung over him. He walked through a poisonous rain. And yet! He breathed deeply as though the air were clear. He walked as though the sun shone and sun rays danced around the corner in front of him.

It's not going to be easy.

The doctor needed a clinic and assistants. His plump figure radiated energy and unflinching confidence. He'd already entered the future and was busy equipping it.

I think that's the way it must have been. There are no notes in the files. All the same, I can hear the story develop.

I can see the streets in Cologne. Ugly, hard streets and glossy windows. I'd prefer my story to leave these streets and travel out into the forest. I'd prefer it to cycle along narrow roads. Daddy has pictures from Germany. I love those pictures. There's a castle deep in the heart of the German forest. Sababurg, it says on the back of the card. Sleeping Beauty once slept there.

That's where I'd like my story to reach on its wanderings

along country roads. And they'd be there, along with the story: Daddy, Mummy, Aunt Tilly, the doctor from Prague. What are they but figments of the imagination? Dreamers. People like that don't walk on a street in Cologne. They don't send in their tax returns and they don't buy bread at the co-op. They belong in Sababurg Castle.

Daddy puts away the picture. The world put an end to stories a long time ago, he says.

I don't believe him. If it were true, why would he save the picture?

Mummy doesn't believe him either. She has me with her in her bed. Her bed forms part of the land of fairy tales. She caresses my hair.

I feel her hand and wonder about the fairy tales. There's a small pond below Sababurg Castle. The doctor sits there on the edge of the pond with his feet in the water-lillies and gazes with curiousity at an ugly little duckling.

It doesn't matter what one looks like, Mummy says suddenly. One can look like anything.

Not like anything!

Almost, she says. Don't mind what others say.

I cuddle up and bury myself inside her. I mind. Everyone minds.

One can have a green tuft in one's hair. She talks about what is right. She talks about what is right as though it were a person. A person who is right. She doesn't ask what one looks like. One can walk around with holes in one's shoes or live in a house in which the windows fall out. That doesn't matter.

How are we supposed to know?

That's the simplest of all, she says. Everyone knows what is right and wrong.

But if they're mistaken? Imagine if you're mistaken!

Is that what you think?

She pulls the quilt higher up and kisses me on the forehead.

We can make mistakes. We can do wrong. The greatest wrongs of all are done in the name of what is right.

No, she says. We know when we do wrong. The wicked know that as well.

At that very moment I see the doctor from Prague. He half runs up a stairs. Right in the center of Cologne they've built this set of stairs that never seems to end. It disappears up amongst glossy windows and dirty clouds.

You must convince them.

One of the doctor's friends tries to keep pace with him.

There are those who doubt.

I don't.

The doctor's friend managed to catch the doctor's coat from behind and stop him.

Those who doubt must be won over.

The doctor pulls himself free and shouts a few words in Czechoslovakian. There'll always be opponents, and they can seldom be won over. They must be conquered.

Those who doubt can be won over, his friend shouted, they must be won over.

He held the doctor's shoulders with his hands and gripped them. I can see the men in front of me standing on the long stairs. I can see how they push and sway and shout. It was serious now. The doctor must convince people if he is to get his clinic.

The doctor pulled himself free. He didn't want to hear about obstacles. He was right and he'd show them. He rushed on and disappeared into the lecture theater at the top.

He gave his lecture among the clouds. He talked about his work in Prague, about the observations he made for many years at the pediatric clinics there. About how he had arranged his observations. He used Latin words and words only doctors understand. *Die cerebralen Bewegungsstörungen im Säuglingsalter.* That's the title of a book I found together with all the other papers and case histories. There are pictures of disabled children, children who seldom learn to creep or walk.

You can see it quite clearly in the children. Even when they're small, you can see it. I don't like that book. I'll never open it again.

The doctor talked for half a day. In front of him sat one hundred wise men and women, the wisest in Cologne. Someone coughed. What had happened was unfortunate, everyone was sorry about what had happened in Prague. Nevertheless, we must ask for substantiating material about the children.

I'm showing you, the doctor said. There are papers, reports.

We've read those, of course. Your reputation has preceded you. But proof? Case histories, documentation?

They're behind in Prague.

Yes, of course, that's true. Sympathetic voices could be heard from the audience. But on the other hand. There's a lot of money involved. . . . You say you can teach all these children to move normally?

Practically.

All of them?

Yes, if no further injury complicates the picture.

Hmm.

And you have nothing more to support this—this supposition?

If it were only a supposition I wouldn't waste your time with it.

His opponents sowed the seeds of doubt, in their gentle and friendly way. People seldom have rows at gatherings like this. They don't stand in the basement and shout beside the boiler the way Daddy does. They snare you with pretended solicitude and a show of being helpful.

One day! The doctor had one day and his lecture. He had seen the outlines of an explanation. It was like a silhouette in the dark. A neurophysiological theory, it's called in the documents. What did they want? No one had been anywhere near, no one had ever been anywhere near this theory.

But was it right?

The outlines can be seen. And what can be seen must be tested and evaluated. The doctor led them on through his lecture. He gave them pictures and let them sit like the shepherds under the first heaven God created. The brain of a child is as complicated as that heaven. What happens in the universe when a streak of light is suddenly extinguished, when a few million suns die out?

You take a ladder, one of those who doubted muttered sarcastically, you climb up and you hang up new suns.

No! You don't light up suns that have gone out, the doctor snapped. You don't replace them as though they were bulbs.

So you can't cure what has happened?

Of course not. You can't repair the damaged parts of a child's brain.

What can you do then?

Open up new paths, make use of other suns.

The doctor collapsed into his lecture chair when they left. Covered in sweat he sat alone against the end wall of the lecture theater. His hands shook and he pressed them against the edge of the desk. Had he really expected victory to be easy?

One of his friends walked slowly back and forth between the rows of benches and regarded the solitary figure. Well, what do you think?

The doctor jumped up from his chair and packed his papers into his briefcase. I won them over. Of course I did. We'll have our pediatric clinic.

§

Aunt Tilly was the first one to see it. She came often that winter. Mummy didn't know how to avoid her. After all,

Aunt Tilly had helped them and now she was entitled to be with them.

Aunt Tilly saw it almost immediately. Her watchful eyes ran over Mummy's stomach.

You're very fat.

Yes, Mummy sighed. She was bigger than when she'd been carrying Lisa.

It's twins, Aunt Tilly said.

Why had no one thought of that! Mummy grew angry. Nonsense, she hissed.

It's twins, Aunt Tilly said stubbornly. You have twins in your family, don't you?

It's not hereditary, Mummy said.

Of course it is, Aunt Tilly said. Fraternal twins are hereditary.

Damn it! Mummy had to go out in the kitchen and put her head under the tap. Why did it have to be Aunt Tilly who said what she herself should have understood long ago! I can't put up with any more of it, she thought. Why couldn't she discover this herself?

It's *my* stomach!

Mummy was so angry she felt a lump in her throat. She talked to Daddy out of earshot of Aunt Tilly.

It's mine! You can't take it away from me. Aunt Tilly will have to go. She comes into our home, she pushes her way into me and now she's trying to occupy my stomach.

Good God, Daddy said.

I'm going to push her out into the snow!

Don't do that, she's helping us.

I don't want her help.

Mummy looked ridiculous. She's completely incapable of swelling up and inspiring fear when she gets angry. She doesn't frighten anyone. Her short legs had sort of shrunk under her huge stomach.

I've seen pictures of pregnant women. They look as though they're turned in on themselves and are sort of silently rejoicing over the state they find themselves in. Pictures like that are taken by men, she says. She herself was fuddled, always fuddled and sweating with red streaks across her stomach. She wished she and her stomach were somewhere else, but most of all she wished Aunt Tilly were somewhere else.

You look like a toad, Daddy said.

He laughed but while he was laughing he put his hand on his back. He had a pain there.

Ouch! he said.

I hope it hurts, Mummy said murderously.

Daddy's backache was a revenge for the furniture and Aunt Tilly. Mummy isn't the sort who tries to get even, she's not the sort who accumulates revenge. But so much had become dreary, so dreadfully dreary. She needed to be left in peace, she needed to feel she had something that was hers alone. She glared at Daddy and her nose stuck out like a little spike from her fuddled face.

§

A new disaster struck Daddy, far worse than the boiler. One day the roof leaked. Rain and slushy snow attacked with undiminished strength. Nature refused to regard their house as approved. When the water had been stopped underneath, it began to run above. They had challenged superior forces. They should have given up.

Daddy leased a tarpaulin. They couldn't afford to repair the roof. He climbed up and managed to pull up the heavy tarpaulin with a rope. And up there, just when he had laid out the tarpaulin and was balanced on the ridge, he had an attack of lumbago.

He couldn't move. They had to call the fire brigade to get him down.

Almost everything that happened around this time seems ridiculous. But I think it's true. They simply couldn't manage. You should see them, I say to myself. If only you knew.

I think things like that fairly often because out there, beyond the house and the garden, everything was different. When Daddy typed on his typewriter out there, it sounded like a machine gun. He wrote like a machine gun and I think he thought like one. No doubt about it. People were talking about his plays. He was interviewed on TV and talked about workers who couldn't breathe. They had dust in their lungs. Once a cabinet minister rang him up and asked about the workers. Beautiful women spoke to him in squeaky voices and wanted to know how he did it. He wrote so beautifully about the poor workers.

Mummy was the same. She'd made clothes for the Beatles. In her sleep she knew everything about fabrics and textile factories and accounting. Even sharp-eyed bank managers became a little uneasy in her presence. She saw through them, saw the figures they were hiding.

§

Daddy whimpered about the pain in his back.

Just a little kindness is all I need, Daddy said and sank down with his backache on a pile of cushions.

I'm not kind, Mummy said.

You could try, Daddy said. It's a matter of training.

I think it's going to be twins, Mummy said.

Good God!

Stop saying good God to everything!

Daddy regarded her with curiosity. Her stomach had a new significance. It had already begun to live an independent life. It required respect and care. One had to show it courtesy and open doors for it.

But now! Wasn't it even more swollen than before? Mummy's stomach swelled out and Mummy grew small. She became an accessory, a fragile collection of bones and stubbornness.

The stomach put itself to bed. Daddy didn't say a word. He went on staring. The stomach filled Mummy's half of the bed. Beneath it she struggled for somewhere for herself. She refused to be regarded as an accessory. She wanted to be the principal figure.

Daddy got up on his knees. He listened with the empty toilet paper roll that evening. It took time. He had to listen in a new way now.

It was like hunting for submarines, he explained later. Your ear becomes a probe, you drag carefully through the depths down there. You hear something but it might be echoes. The stomach bubbles, its bed releases sounds.

Furthest down beneath the navel he heard the first sound, the well-known sound he had already captured. One hundred and thirty-seven beats. But the second sound, was there a second sound?

He dragged his probe upwards. You have to be silent, so silent that nothing else can be heard. You mustn't even breathe. No one must breathe in the room. Suddenly he stiffened. Was there something there? Down at the bottom under dark shadows. The new sound is never what you expect it to be. It's not like the first sound.

Do you hear anything?

Mummy puffed and had to take a breath. Daddy looked up, frowning. Who's talking? Oh yes, of course, she was there. In the room too. Well, she'd have to be quiet and stop breathing.

I must breathe, she said.

You're disturbing me.

He was leaning over her again, concentrating. You have to open your senses while the proble moves around in circles, round and round the suspected point. That was what was important, switching sense organs to receive new and unexpected ranges of perception.

There! A weak and altogether different sound. He lay as though he were part of her and searched for his watch amongst the bedclothes. Shine the light on the watch!

What can you hear?

Quiet! He counted. It could still be an echo from the child further down. But it wasn't an echo.

Oh. He let go of the watch and rolled over on his side amongst the cushions. A different beat, a more uncertain beat, slower, like the weak breathing of a young bird. One hundred twenty-three beats. Two lives!

What is it? Mummy turned towards him.

Probably a twin, he said, and stared at the ceiling.

§

It was me!

From now on I'm the main figure in this story. That's one of the reasons I'm writing it while the others are asleep. They don't really want to acknowledge me as the main figure. They'd be hurt and force their way into my story, they'd stand in front of me, they'd throw shadows over my memories and make me a sort of reason for what happened. They were so proud. I was the reason they felt so proud and remarkable.

Almost all parents are like that. Self-centered. When Daddy falls asleep at night he sighs and says that now the whole world is falling asleep.

They needed me. First of all they held happiness in their arms when I was born. Then they needed me to tie themselves to each other. A child was going to help them to straighten out their confused and crooked lives.

For the first time I really existed. On the desk in front of me I build up a theater. I push aside the files and put the rabbit in my rucksack. The stage is wide open and I step out onto it. The baby! The main part everyone's been waiting for but nobody recognizes. I dance and I sing. I'm the infant prodigy who glides forward. I do what no one else can do. The audience stands up and excitement runs through it like uneasy waves. I can see the doctor from Prague out there, the doctor who wants to use my body.

And Mummy and Daddy who are going to become more complete human beings thanks to their child.

They shout and protest that I've stolen the main part from them. Not until it's too late will they discover that they've been turned into stone.

You thought you had something, didn't you? You increased and multiplied. You were so satisfied with yourself that you wanted to make more of you. And I, Asa, was going to be your eternal life. That's why I turn you into stone.

You're unfair, I'm unfair.

I hear Granny's voice. She's approaching the story, I sense her here, her smell, the feeling that surrounds her. She sits at my desk and I cry. She hugs me and my tears wet the lace on her blouse. Everything about her is so fine, her features are so delicate and her eyes once cried over a thousand sorrows.

Her presence calms me. She clears things up. She explains. We don't choose our existence. We mustn't blame our parents. Not too severely, at any rate. There are people who make a living out of ridiculing their parents, their mothers, mostly, because they're easiest to get at.

Granny has soft, narrow hands and they feel their way across my face. Being born is like . . . she searches for an image . . . it's like falling into a big pit. Everyone falls into the pit and everyone tries to get out of it.

We can blame others. That's the easiest. But almost no one can forgive.

Your Mummy and Daddy . . . she starts to say something as though she had an explanation. The explanation for everything. She speaks so clearly you can hear every syllable. She doesn't blur what she says like the others. Mummy always says two things at the same time and has a third on its way out.

Your Mummy and Daddy . . . she stops there. Granny puts her head on one side and suddenly begins to laugh.

You must see the ridiculous side of it, the forgiving and the ridiculous side.

We laugh together. That's the best of all, laughing together with her while the tears roll out like tiny balls from the corners of her eyes.

I'm the main figure in this story.

Of course, dear Asa.

The laughter dies out. But small titters hang on and scamper along the floor. Just imagine! Daddy found me that evening with his searching probe. I was pushed aside. That's why it was difficult to find me.

My sister lay in the center of Mummy's stomach. I imagine her like an octopus, a big brooding octopus with its arms swaying in the currents and the tides. Octopuses have yellow eyes and a beak in the centre of their heads. She eats and grows and everything around her is soft and warm.

But I'm being pushed upwards. There isn't room enough for me. I had to live in the attic. Up there I lay crookedly, turned in the wrong direction, and I must have spent a lot of my first year like that. No room to move, the roof pressing down on me with Mummy's sharp thorax on my back.

And the constant lack of food! Berit had a big, marvelous placenta that gave her all the nourishment she needed. I got scarcely a corner of it. When she'd gulped down all she wanted I had to search for crumbs under the table. No wonder my heart ticked weakly. No wonder my brain was like a small blue jellyfish. No wonder my twisted legs were as thin as old spaghetti you throw out with the slops. No wonder I demand to be allowed to play my part, the main part.

Dear Asa!

Granny makes an abrupt movement with her hand. I don't know what this movement means, but a current of air carries her scent to me. She buys perfume on planes. She takes foam baths. Daddy says she smells first class and girls' school.

How charming! I can hear their voices and their delighted cries while I desperately try to create a little more space for myself. Just a little more space and a little more food! But I don't have enough strength, I can't manage it!

Twins, isn't that sweet! They poked about in their own delight. Like when you look at piglets. How they push and shove and root around. Cheerful cries criss-cross through the air while the smallest piglet, the one that's going to die, can't make it. It'd be better if the sow bit it to death straight off.

Asa! Granny tries gently to lead the story in another direction. Have you forgotten the laughter?

Daddy was the most ridiculous. Filled up over his ears with his new importance. Twins make you interesting. You attract attention, you can strew silly jokes around you. Daddy saw himself with a cigar in his hand waiting in the maternity ward. Well, what is it? Ha ha, it's an entire flock.

They already spoke of The Twins. They still do. But I'm not a twin. I'm Asa!

Daddy's eyes were shiny and his mouth looked foolish when he'd been drinking wine. From now on, he said, we must think of everything as duplicated. Everything will be doubled, love, sorrow, children's allowances. Twins can be sold for research.

Mummy put her hand on his mouth.

Researchers love twins.

Identical twins, Mummy said. Only identical twins.

They experiment with twins, Daddy said.

Be quiet! Don't talk like that.

Women have no sense of humor, Daddy says. They never play, they seldom dare make fun of themselves. They're so serious.

I don't like you talking like that, Mummy said.

Ah, he hadn't really thought of selling the twins for research. Not really.

There are so many other markets where children can be

sold. You can make an asset out of them. You can tell a funny story about your children and make an asset out of them, the glasses clink, your friends laugh and you tell them something funny about your children. You sell your children for a laugh.

While I lie there waiting for the thin blood that's never quite enough. My blind eyes need oxygen to see. I'm being strangled!

Mummy could feel anxiety like a push in the back. There's always a risk. Sometimes you can see pictures of quadruplets and quintuplets. They're often born far away. I've seen newspaper pictures from Italy. There people have sextuplets. The newspapers congratulate them. What a sensation! But the children often die. Or there's something wrong with them. I've seen a calf with two heads in a museum.

Daddy couldn't understand Mummy's anxiety. He bathed in his new importance. Strong men have a lot of children. It's a question of virility, he says. The strongest get twins. He stretched his muscles and admired himself as he stood there in his dreadful underpants.

Everything was going well for him. The theater was sold out every night. Everyone wanted to see Daddy's play about the misery of the workers. He made money and he could buy steaks and repair the roof. A chiropractor straightened out his joints. Everything was wonderful. Doesn't one have a right to be happy?

One mustn't get bogged down. Mummy overcame her anxiety. Even she could see how her importance increased. Nature had courted her and selected her to play a special part. It makes me angry and jealous to think of her chattering away on the telephone, her happiness at having a new subject to talk about. Just imagine. That she. She!

While my brain wasn't getting enough of her oxygen. Everything was going so well for them, everything was so nice and pleasant. They had no room for me.

§

Not even science had room for me.

Mummy slid and slipped through the snow. A lot of snow had come. It was very cold. She edged her stomach into the warm prenatal clinic.

Everything's fine, the doctor said.

They'd weighed and measured and listened. The doctor clapped her on the stomach.

But there's one problem, the doctor said. A big problem.

Mummy shivered. That sounded ominous.

You're too narrow, the doctor continued. Your pelvis is too narrow.

Oh, Mummy said.

You can't get children out through that pelvis, the doctor said.

How odd, Mummy said.

Not at all, the doctor said. He began to give her a lecture on the human pelvis.

There's just one thing I wonder about, Mummy said.

He wasn't listening. He was a Man of Science and he was showing her a chart.

I wonder, she said again.

What do you wonder? the doctor asked irritably. He didn't like being interrupted.

I already have two children, Mummy said. They were born without any complications. I wonder how they got out. Through my ear maybe?

The doctor began to bark. He just stood there barking. It was something about the case history. Then he told off his nurse, a midwife who became frightened and unhappy. The doctor claimed the case history was incomplete.

Mummy interrupted him again. She dares do things like that. She even dares interrupt doctors.

And there are two of them, she said.

No, the doctor said.

They're twins, Mummy said.

The doctor had been fully occupied with firing off blazing arrows at the midwife. Now he turned on Mummy and looked like a surgeon who likes to operate without anaesthetic.

How do you know there are twins?

My husband listened to them, Mummy said.

Your husband? The doctor looked through the papers and made a fuss. He wanted to get his own back. As far as I can see you're not married.

The children's father, Mummy said.

The child's father, the doctor corrected her.

The children's father, Mummy said, has listened to the children.

And how did he listen?

At that moment Mummy realized she wasn't going to get any help, not the sort of help that might be needed for twins, no advice, nothing.

Well, how did he listen? the doctor repeated.

Through an empty toilet paper roll, she said.

I see, the doctor said, and looked out over his landscape of expensive medical equipment. I see. He turned away and shot off an order towards the door. Next!

Mummy stumbled out of the prenatal clinic. Climbing the slope up from the door she slipped and ended up sitting in a snow drift. She rubbed her face with snow, her humiliated, burning face.

The unhappy midwife came after her. She helped Mummy up from the snow drift. You shouldn't sit in the snow. You'll catch cold.

The doctor glared out at them between the curtains at the window of the clinic. The midwife gave Mummy a hug.

What a turn things can take, she muttered, and disappeared back into the clinic.

§

The doctor from Prague stumbled down the long stairs. Buses roared past outside in the dusk. Worn-out shoes hurried across the cobblestones. His shirt stuck, ice-cold with old sweat, across his back.

It was the sort of day when you step out in front of a bus. Screaming brakes, people who look away to avoid seeing what happened.

He stopped suddenly so that those behind almost knocked him over. He leaned against the front of a building while shadows rushed through his exhausted head.

A darkened world, a state of desperation!

Proof, doctor. You must understand that we need more than we've heard just now.

He took a deep breath. You mustn't show your anguish. Surely they'd heard about his results in Prague.

Yes, they'd heard and they'd read about them, they nodded in agreement. But they'd heard other things as well. That the children suffered. That the doctor mistreated the children.

He stood on a street in Cologne, sunk in coming defeats when a voice sought his attention. What's wrong? Aren't you well?

A white-haired man, one of those who had listened to his lecture, emerged from the hurrying, stumbling flow of human beings. The doctor rubbed his eyes with the back of his hand. He looked up. It was like seeing a picture emerge in a photographer's dark-room.

You're worried, the white-haired man said.

A pale necklace of street lamps lit up at that moment. More rain was on the way. You could see it from the lamps, the doctor thought. Damp air absorbs the light.

An outstanding lecture, the white-haired man said.

I can see them stand there. I see a shower of sparks. Like when an electric cable strikes the earth. Plus and minus meet. That's where my story is born.

I and the doctor from Prague!

A lot of people who are interested, the white-haired man said.

How many? the doctor asked.

Enough. I think I can guarantee that you'll get your clinic.

Chapter Five

Winter sharpened its teeth. It ripped at those who were unprotected and brought down those who were old. Winter moved on. What was left of it murmured along the gutters.

Mummy stood on the steps. She had the front door key in her hand. For the rest of her life she'll carry with her the details of that moment. Lisa stood a few steps lower down. Mummy had tied a lovely blue bow in Lisa's hair.

Sunday. A quarter past one. Mummy put the key in the lock to lock the front door. The weather had changed. First it had been windy with a lot of sunshine which poured down over the roofs. Now big snow flakes came floating on the wind. Lisa put her hands above her head in a vain attempt to protect her bow.

It had been one of those wonderful mornings. Beyond sleep and the warmth of her bed, Mummy had heard Daddy rummage about. He kissed her on the ear when he said goodbye and flew off to the north of Sweden. Patrick had gone to fish through the spring ice with his father.

Mummy lay in bed all morning and let sleep and wakefulness fight it out. She heard the church bells. She remembers the church bells in particular. She never goes to church. But she wouldn't miss the church bells for anything. She's about as much of a churchgoer as a farmer from the south of Sweden, Daddy says. A farmer who goes out on the veranda, stretches his arms, listens to the bells and then goes back to bed again. Religious as a Swede, Daddy says.

Now she and Lisa were finally on their way into town to

look at a women's lib exhibition. She turned the key and as she did so she felt the warm fluid run along her legs. She'd never been so afraid before. She remembers that clearly. You sort of become petrified, she says. All your movements stop. You sink down. She's tried to describe it. But she says that no matter how she describes it it's much worse, not the feeling but rather the sudden absence of feeling. The fluid ran. It was six weeks too early and it was a disaster.

I can see her standing outside the door. Her hand still on the key. Lisa standing three steps lower down. Hurry up, Mummy! My bow. . . . Lisa is suddenly silent. She's six years old. Old enough to see when someone is ill and dying with fear.

Mummy opened the door and went in. She walked with straight legs as though doing so might prevent or lessen what had happened. She was open. The protection was gone. You can do things even when you're afraid. You can do practical things, talk with your mouth and move your hands. The fear catches you in the throat. Nevertheless, you do things.

Lisa helped her to pack a small suitcase with essentials. Mummy telephoned. First she telephoned to the north of Sweden but it was impossible to get in touch with Daddy. She telephoned a friend and made arrangements for Lisa. She telephoned for two taxis.

Mummy explained. Lisa stood with the little suitcase in her arms. Her bow hung down over her ears. She was a little calf on narrow legs looking on when the cow falls and kicks.

What a good girl you are, Mummy said.

Lisa let go of the suitcase and hugged her.

They went off in different directions. They waved to each other from the taxis as long as they could see each other.

Mummy stood outside the maternity hospital and rang the bell. Heavy snow flakes struck her in the face. She'd put her suitcase on the ground. She stood with her arms over her stomach, incapable of protecting her face.

The rest is medical case histories.

Daddy got hold of copies of them. I have them in piles in front of me on the desk. Some of them went crookedly into the copying machine and have black edges. They look like the black edges on mourning cards. So many case histories! You could wallpaper the entire house with them.

Admitted for amniotic fluid discharge at 1:45 p.m. it says at the top of the first page of the journal.

§

This wasn't Mummy's hospital. She'd had her other children in the north. She didn't feel at home here. A bad hospital! I can't tell you how many times she repeated that.

It was the hospital's fault, she says.

No, Daddy says. It wasn't as bad as that.

What happened after was the hospital's fault, she says.

An old, worn-out hospital with a lot of moaning hidden behind the barrage of foreign words they use in the case histories. But the view! On the very top of the rocky hill the wards floated high above the city. You could see forests and sun, water and roofs.

Daddy shambled in from the corridors and the lifts. He'd arrived with the last evening plane. Department 70, Ward 5, they told him at the reception. Mummy was already inserted and numbered.

She lay quite still in the sunset. Nothing had changed since midday. Fear still caught at her above the throat and her eyes were shining. She wasn't permitted to move.

Daddy sat on the edge of the bed and tried to find comforting words. Everything would be all right.

She was wide open. Her children lay unprotected.

He understood that.

Six weeks!

Don't worry, he said. Try not to worry. A lot of children are born too early.

She nodded. His presence helped. It helped a little. And his unwavering confidence.

They've postponed the birth, she said and managed to produce a smile. They'd given her something to delay it.

Good, he said. Isn't modern technology marvelous. You just pick the date you want. They can do anything.

Is that good?

Of course it's good. He almost managed to persuade her with his optimism.

They whispered to each other. They didn't want to disturb the other women. What about the twins? Had they been acknowledged?

Almost. A number of trainee midwives had been there and listened and felt. They'd heard two hearts. But the trainees weren't good enough. Not until two days later would the doctors discover the twins.

You can see that in the case history. Somebody's added a note afterwards. X-rays required. The doctors are quite helpless without their equipment. Duplex, somebody else's hand has written. And furthest down at the bottom of the page, in the margin, they've put me. A marginal child. TW II, it says. Me, Asa, Twin II.

§

Daddy left. He looked satisfied. Mummy was in good hands now. The children were secure. Everyone could breathe a sigh of relief. He waved to her from the doorway as he went.

That's fine, she thought. He's reassured. That's fine for him. Carefully she got out of bed and walked over to the window. She'd hoped to catch a glimpse of him down there. But you couldn't see the exit from the window. He was going to take the morning plane back to Norrland again. Just for a few days. The twins are growing and you're doing fine.

The other women regarded her with sympathy. But they were too far away. One is enclosed, one can't break out. She walked over the lavatory. Inside she held on to a shining steel tube on the wall above the WC.

It was an unusual WC. There was a shower in the bowl. You pressed a button and the shower washed you clean. She pressed the button for a long time.

§

She washed herself clean and enjoyed it. She flushed water from a shower installed in the dirty bowl straight up into her unprotected womb. What trust! In that damned hospital!

It was the hospital's fault! Her voice goes out of control when she blames the hospital. Evening after evening they've gone over this again and again. When they think I'm asleep they start. Her voice is sharp and piercing in a way it never is otherwise. Someone's fault? They're talking about me. I'm someone's fault.

I put the pillow over my head. But I hear them anyway.

It wasn't really the shower, Daddy says.

Of course it was, Mummy says. A dirty, disgusting hospital.

Wait a minute, Daddy says.

But she won't wait. Dirt everywhere. Slut's wool in the corridors outside the operating theater. In the maternity ward all the newborn babies had infected navels.

Not our babies, Daddy says.

She grows furious. He won't believe her. But she knows. She's found out everything about the hospital, she says. About the filth. In the ophthalmic department they didn't even have a changing room. The staff had to change in the lavatory before they went into the operating theater.

You weren't in the ophthalmic ward, he says.

You don't believe me, she says.

It's not that.

What is it then? She talks about the Sachsska Children's Hospital, the annex where we were transferred later. The chief physician at the Sachsska Hospital . . .

Can't you stop!

. . . The chief physician at the Sachsska Hospital boasted that they had the lowest cost per patient. Their cost was only half the average cost. Don't you see what that means?

The accusations become a sort of game. A mystery game, Daddy says. Even if a lot of what she says is true, he refuses to agree with her. After all, he's collected the documents that make up the case history. They've been explained to him by doctors. Skilful doctors he trusts.

The doctors protect each other, Mummy says. Of course they do. Ignorant and smug, they try to get the best of everything. They tramp around in their hospital infections. They demand huge sums of money for research to get rid of it. If they only allocated a fraction of the money to improved cleaning!

It's important to be rational, Daddy says.

I *am* rational.

He waves the documents in front of her. Why doesn't she listen.

Because there's nothing to listen to.

According to the case history they didn't make any mistakes. No major mistakes.

She takes them from him. She pulls them out of his hands. Anyone who wants to see can see. There it is, amongst all the strange words. E-coli.

I know, Daddy says.

In their lungs. Their lungs were filled with coli bacteria! It's disgusting.

These things happen sometimes, Daddy says.

Where did the bacteria come from?

Daddy tries to sound scientific. He thinks that'll help.

Excrement from the fetus. You can see it here. He points. Meconium-colored amniotic fluid, it says.

Why do they do it? Mummy says.

Because . . . Daddy hesitates.

Why?

No one knows for sure. They probably become stressed. They release their excrement and that, in turn, triggers the birth.

So the coli bacteria came from them, Mummy says.

No, the fetus' excrement is sterile.

Where do they come from? She sounds more frantic than ever. I press the pillows down harder over my head. I don't want to listen and I can't sleep.

You know, Mummy says. I know. The bacteria came from me. From the shower.

Perhaps, Daddy says. But they might have come from the actual delivery as well.

They let me lie open, Mummy says. Nowhere else is a woman let lie open more than twenty-four hours.

Daddy sighs.

You see! That damned hospital and those damned explanations that aren't a damned bit better because they're in Latin.

I scream. I don't want to hear them any longer. I scream to silence them. They run up the stairs to my room. They try to comfort me but they can't.

§

Mummy used the shower. She exchanged a few words with the other women. But there was no real conversation. She couldn't break out of her fear.

She lay down on the bed and waited for the disaster to be completed.

You suspect yourself. That's the first thing. That's why you must blame others. The suspicion sits there on your shoulder. It lies waiting on the bedside table.

You lie there defenselessly. Others judge. Others stand at the end of the bed and judge. You listen with growing anxiety. What did the doctor say? Didn't she hear a change in his tone of voice?

You lie absolutely still. Mustn't disturb the babies in there. No stress. That's the way you talk to yourself while disaster is already going beserk inside you.

She really had longed for these days. The days in the maternity ward are delightful, filled with women's talk and self-reflection that needs no excuses. Oh, how she had longed!

She turned and twisted in her bed. She listened for the sound of the hospital. Everyone in the ward slept quietly. What had she done wrong? The fetuses protested, her body didn't acknowledge them, they were rejected. She slept uneasily now and then and longed for Granny. But Granny lives in another town and couldn't come.

It was Aunt Tilly who came. The next morning she came, an unlikely apparition with her arms full of boxes of chocolate, a thermos, and tulips she'd bought at half price. She forced her way in before the visiting hours, threatened the ward sister that she'd report her, she hung up her bags and tore around the ward with a sizzling spate of words.

Aunt Tilly inspected. With devastating instinct she measured the quality of the hospital. She wasn't satisfied with what she saw.

She hunted out a few smoking orderlies from the entrance hall and got them to fetch vases. She offered everyone chocolates while she explained how important Daddy was.

He was so important that he had to travel to Norrland and that was why Aunt Tilly was going to move into our house, to take care of Lisa and keep things in order.

Just for a few days, she said.

Thanks, Mummy whispered.

Aunt Tilly sank down into the visitor's chair. She let

loose new torrents of words. Mummy closed her eyes without really listening. It was something about men.

Men break into the maternity ward, Aunt Tilly said. They refuse to give up. They practice breathing together with their women, they train for the delivery and then when the time comes they . . .

What? Mummy whispered.

I'm talking about men, Aunt Tilly said. They're envious of us. They suspect we have rich emotions. They want what's ours. Everything. They already have the executive jobs and political power. But they're not satisfied.

I think they should participate in the delivery, Mummy said. She grew irritable.

They take over, Aunt Tilly said. They break in to steal women's emotions, they assault the maternity wards and soon it'll be the men who do the lying-in.

Now she had to go.

What's the chief physician called, she asked?

I don't know, Mummy said.

I'll ring the chief physician, Aunt Tilly said. You must find out how long you're going to lie here like that.

Don't, Mummy said.

Aunt Tilly bent over her. Maybe I can have you moved to another hospital.

No!

This hospital isn't good. Everyone knows that.

Mummy couldn't listen to her anymore. Anyway her plan was mad and meaningless. It's not a question of choice.

I can arrange it so that you're moved, Aunt Tilly muttered.

Please, don't you understand, I don't want to, it's not possible, not even you can do that.

Aunt Tilly looked hurt. She's part of the heart of the city. She knows all the tricks. She's always first in any queue. Even if she's the last to arrive.

She was born with the city and every cobblestone was

laid for her sake. She worked for the city and when the city was thrifty she was thrifty. Envelopes were always used twice. You turned them inside out.

She keeps track of the hospitals and everything else that's important. Like when you should become ill and where you should go. There are people who sit waiting for five hours in the casualty department. Never Aunt Tilly.

She always gets a sudden pain. Even if she's had the pain for weeks. Suddenly she's in pain. And it's a Saturday morning. The Friday evening drunks have been bandaged and ordinary people haven't yet woken up and discovered that they're ill.

You have to keep track of the short cuts in the city, Aunt Tilly says, the short cuts the authorities have forgotten to close off. If you want to survive. The meek are the first to go to the wall.

Aunt Tilly left Mummy. She charged out to the taxis with her handbag full of transport vouchers from the Social Welfare. God only knows where she got hold of them. Out there it was spring and Monday morning.

§

The next three days are almost completely wiped out. Fear was their focal point and all around there were checks, voices, and routines. Those days are almost completely gone. Left is the sense of loss over what didn't happen. The first labor pains came on the morning of the third day. It was half past five.

It's painful, Mummy says. But one forgets. In some odd way one forgets almost immediately.

That's the way it had been before. But not this time. Nothing was the same as before and nothing was recognizable. Everything inside her became cramp and panic.

She remembers the bed rolling out, the corridors, the rapid footsteps. Something was beginning to go wrong. She saw without seeing. The pain tore her apart. It twisted her like a rag. She had to say goodbye. She had to meet Daddy and say goodbye.

He arrived and stood beside her bed. They were in some sort of anteroom shining with the usual fluorescent lights and steel. He talked and he squeezed her hand. She wanted to say her final words but couldn't.

The pain stood in the way. Nothing came from her except a plaintive moaning. Daddy was there. She knew that but she couldn't reach out to him. What would happen to Lisa? She thought of the blue bow. How silly that she should think of that now! The wrinkled bow. And Daddy was so bad at ironing.

Do something! Why did they refuse to help her?

They should have done a Caesarean, Mummy says.

We can't blame them, Daddy says.

§

No?

He dives down in the case history to show her something. He riffles through the documents. There was no reason, no indications, he says. There was nothing that indicated a Caesarean.

But she knew. All her body knew. After all, she'd had children before. The doctors had never had children. The pain wasn't a natural pain. Not even for childbirth was it natural. It tore her apart inside. It came in jackboots and stamped on the children and on everything that fed them and kept them alive.

There was one thing she managed to say. They must give her something for the pain. The pain can be relieved by an anaesthetic in the spine. She whispered it and she shouted it. She was promised.

Someone promised, a nurse, a midwife. She doesn't remember who. The anaesthetists were to start work at eight o'clock. She'd get it then. The promise was a hook. She hung up the rest of her moaning, bawling life on that hook.

You have to accept the way things are. If you're going to give birth you'd better do it during office hours.

The pains were so bad now that they couldn't get any worse. But they got worse. They crossed the limit for what was possible. It was eight o'clock. Now! She saw them approach. At last!

Spinal anaesthetic, she slurred.

Not possible, they said.

You promised.

No we didn't.

You tricked me!

They tried to calm her down. They patted her on the cheek. They explained. A spinal anaesthetic can only be given for a normal delivery.

They tricked her! In a calculated and cold-blooded way they tricked her. That damned hospital!

If only I could remember those hours! The disaster. The cramp blocks everything. The blood flow weakens, the oxygen supply dies out. Daddy pokes about in his scientific insights. It may be true that the oxygen supply died out, he says. The flow of blood through the placenta decreases. But that needn't be the hospital's fault. We don't know.

Mummy knows.

If only she could die. She longed to die. If only she could faint. But the pain was as cunning as those green beings out there. The pain kept her conscious. Enough for her to feel it and scream.

They pulled her down the corridors. To the operating theater, for safety's sake. Daddy was sent off. He wasn't allowed to enter the operating theater. He stood in the waiting room. Everything would be all right. He was still convinced. He riffled through the sort of magazines that lie around waiting rooms. Gossip magazines. The sort of magazines considered suitable for those who wait.

He tried to imagine how a waiting father-to-be should behave. Waiting fathers-to-be also have parts written for them. They're supposed to be on the verge of collapse.

Life's big moment is at hand. They're supposed to have cigars in their breast pockets, to say crazy things and to have sweaty palms.

The proper atmosphere refused to come. He walked around a little, smoked, and looked through the magazines. He read articles about missionaries and magnets. It's only in waiting rooms you read articles like that. The thing to do is to have magnets put in the soles of your shoes. If you do, you'll live until you die, it said.

Mummy remembers less. She remembers the blood, the blood and the raging roar that shattered the entire world into fragments. Someone called for blood. She remembers that. And she remembers the answer. There's no time to check.

Berit emerged first. She sailed out in a nose dive. She's always best at diving, at swimming, at dancing. It was half past eight when they rushed off with her.

I didn't want to. I refused. There was so much space in there! It was so marvelous to be on my own! But they wouldn't let me alone. They dug about in Mummy. They fished around. I didn't have the right position. They got hold of one foot.

Mummy saw me through rivers of sweat and tears. You're forced out. You can't lie in there in that big warm space. She saw my foot stick out. It was blue as a blueberry. They got hold of my other foot and they held on. Can a baby live with feet like that? With a color like that? They pulled me out feet first and rushed off with me at once.

On the reanimation table I'd come to life. I'd be shaken to life, sucked to life, I'd be made to breathe and pulsate and fight my way into life. Asa is a fighter! Daddy keeps saying that. Life must be conquered. You must fight your way to it.

They have tables. They give points to those who are to live and those who are to die. The tables consist of squares on white paper. It's called Apgar. Heart rate: None. Breathing: None. The put an X in the boxes. For every X you get a point. Those who have no points die. I have the Apgar tables here and I can look through them. They lie among all the other documents Daddy has collected.

There's something in between. After one minute, at thirty-nine minutes past eight, I lay on the reanimation table and somewhere beside me my sister Berit kicked. She got full points almost at once. I'm fed up with her points. She's best in school. She's the one who scores in basketball.

No reactions, it says in my box. Pale blue. Limp. You get no points for things like that. I was in between. I got three points.

For some reason my heart beat.

Mummy heard the last cramp echo away in her body. She heard the sounds of the hospital behind closed doors. Suddenly the room was empty.

They forgot her.

I've seen it happen in films, in a comic film with Monty Python. The doctors have tried their new equipment. One of the units says *plip.* Another says *plop.* When the units had finished plipping and plopping and the baby had been delivered everyone disappeared.

Daddy almost died laughing when he watched the film on video.

Mummy lay there alone. What am I going to do now, she thought? How am I going to get out of here? At first she didn't dare move. After a while she felt her body gingerly with her hands. Out there somewhere in those rooms! What were they doing with her babies?

Later, she didn't know how much later, the door was opened and a nurse came in. The nurse was going to put things in order.

I'm in the way, Mummy thought. I'm probably a nuisance. They want to air the place and clean up and here I lie and make the place untidy. That's the way she thought the first second or so but then she pulled herself together and asked the obvious question.

What are they?

What do you mean? the nurse said. She'd become involved in one of the pieces of plipping equipment.

I was wondering what they are?

Oh, the nurse said. Don't you know? Hasn't anyone told you?

§

Daddy stood outside a pane of glass. He saw me for the first time. Berit and I and other newly born babies lie in shining glass boxes. He wasn't allowed to touch us. He wasn't allowed to breathe near us.

Mummy longed to cry. The nurse was trying to be kind. She wanted to comfort Mummy, who had been forgotten.

You mustn't be sad, the nurse said.

I'm not sad, Mummy said.

You mustn't be sad that it was twins, the kind nurse continued. It's not so bad. It doesn't really mean such a lot of work.

I'm happy, Mummy said, and felt altogether empty inside.

You should be glad it's girls, the nurse said. There's nothing as much trouble as twin boys.

Everything went well, Daddy said. He placed the palm of his hand against the pane of glass and bent forward when they pointed. There! There are your children.

I don't think he thought so much about it. Neither of them thought or knew. They were empty the way people are empty when they've lost something. Nice that it's over! That was as far as he thought.

§

At the same time the doctor from Prague sat down behind a big desk. He was wearing a white coat. They'd given him his clinic and the shining eyes of mothers were reflected from the desktop.

They brought him their children the way the wise men brought their gifts. They shook their children who had twisted legs. Help us! Is there any cure? I see them and beyond them I see others waiting, children with crutches, children in wheelchairs.

§

I lay in my glass box and was given the oxygen I couldn't take in myself. I lay there with a tube in my nose because I couldn't eat. After five minutes I had six points. Six on the Apgar. Life was a pursuer and soon it would catch up with me. But after twenty-four hours I still had blue legs.

I got through! Daddy's made a note beneath the points. Ninety-two per cent, he's written. The statistical chance for me was now ninety-two per cent.

Chapter Six

They practiced understanding. Particularly Mummy. You know almost nothing. You're as unprotected as a child in an open womb. You feel as stupid as the stupid pupil in the class.

You can see it with your own eyes. You see that the child you've given birth to is balanced on the edge of life. But you don't know. You can't get behind the words. What do the doctor's words mean? *Norm config., hepar and lien not palp.* it says in Berit's case history. *Umbilicus and inguer norm.*

You tell yourself you must practice seeing things more clearly. You must become alert. You concentrate all your senses and all your capacity on listening. You listen to intonations again and again from every possible angle. Are there any gaps? Is there something they're not saying?

Mummy made her way forward through an underground tunnel. We were transferred to the children's hospital and we had to go through a long tunnel to get there. Mummy thinks of herself as underground that first week. Constantly on her way through the tunnel with her senses opened underground for signals nobody else could perceive.

They could come to see us. But only at specific times. They had to change clothes and pass through air locks. We had trouble keeping the right temperature, we had trouble eating, we had trouble with almost everything.

That's normal enough in itself, the doctor said. Babies born so early have difficulties.

They took photographs. Daddy stands in a white coat, holding me in his arms.

How small she is. Almost nothing to hold. One must be careful when one holds beings as small as that.

I weighed one thousand nine hundred and forty grammes. Less than two pints of milk. I looked like a fetus, transparent, you could almost see my eyes through my eyelids. My legs were spindly. I was so thin that I looked as though I didn't have any behind. Mummy says they loved me anyway.

Berit was getting on better. She was rosier. She weighed more.

They looked at us and felt us. They came with all their longing and all their hope and there, inside the air lock, so much had to take place during those brief meetings. Love bounced back. Their longing moved sleepily through an underground tunnel.

Were there any gaps, any gaps the doctors missed.

§

Spring danced in across the city. It already sat in the parks and longed for summer. I'd been taken out of the glass box. But that was as far as I'd got. I didn't get out into the spring.

Mummy went to the hospital every day. She was always there. It was almost as though she were bothering them. She walked up the small path that wound its way up to the children's hospital. She stood by the stone balustrade and looked out over the precipice and the water below.

She couldn't avoid seeing and feeling, although so much was sad. Now, afterwards, I'm there with her as she stands by the stone balustrade. My nose is damp. I'm the spring that nudges against her with its nose and tries to attract her attention. There's no avoiding the light and what's new. When spring arrives the streets become broader. The wind is wild and flighty and picks up the dust. You shiver and you sweat and you creep into a corner of the garden. Snowdrops grow in just that corner and there you can sit and entice spring to part with the first of her heat.

Mummy watched but she seldom laughed. The two small cots stood empty at home. She'd sewn and arranged things. And how she could sew! What delightful colours! Welcome home! She'd imagined our homecoming as a caress of colours and the softest of fabrics. She'd chosen the best cots, the sort of cots you can't get crushed in. Nothing had been forgotten and now the cots were like empty holes.

They'd considered names. Even when we'd been born they were still uncertain. That's why we were called TW I and TW II in the hospital case histories. Daddy wanted something Nordic. Asa! He thought that sounded strong and healthy.

Mummy wanted Berit. Berit was the name of a girl who, at 16 years of age, had already led a strike at a soap factory in Stockholm. Mummy wanted a girl like that.

Each evening she said goodnight to two empty cots and in the morning the cots were the first thing she saw.

Aunt Tilly came with lots of children's clothes. They made Daddy happy but Mummy didn't want them. She selected a few things, but most of them she threw away. Now *she* was going to do the selecting. Nothing second hand. Nothing at half price. Only the best and most beautiful would do.

Aunt Tilly wasn't allowed to come any more. Not even Mummy's politicals were allowed to come although there was more injustice than ever in the world.

Mummy was like a wounded animal that goes off and hides itself. Daddy saw that. He tried to say things but they weren't the right things.

She wove together her worry and the latest reports from the doctors. The thread she wove of them became thinner and thinner. Daddy didn't want to brood.

We can't get any further, he said.

She searched for new angles, new ways of looking at it. Maybe there was something they hadn't thought of.

He asked her to think about something else. At any rate, to talk about something else. There was no point in pushing uncertainty between them.

She had to talk about it. But who could she talk with?

I talk about it, Daddy said. I'm doing everything I can. But we've reached a point where there's nothing more to say.

You have nothing more to say? She thought he was cold. That he didn't care. Isn't it for precisely moments like this that they had each other? Daddy wasn't up to it all. He fell asleep. How could he sleep so securely?

She walked up the path towards the children's hospital. If only she could enjoy the spring! She went to the hospital for two weeks. Four weeks.

Soon, the doctor said. The children must grow a little and become strong.

How long?

Just two more weeks.

Every day she went to give milk. She had a little milking machine, called Sister Britta's breast pump, and she used it to press out the valuable drops. Soon she'd dry out. She could feel it. Imagine waking every morning when it's time to breast feed your children. Getting up and instead of finding a little living bundle, finding Sister Britta's breast pump waiting for you.

While she was staying at the hospital the times when they'd all milked together had made welcome breaks. She'd taken the lift up under the hospital roof and sat at a long table together with the other women. They sat there in rows and pumped milk. The children needed it. Life needed it.

She liked being at that table. A lot of them talked and were happy. Despite everything. They talked about women who had specialized in doing this. One can make a living from one's own milk. You milk and you sell the milk.

In those days they sold the milk to the Dairy Co-op. There was one door there for human milk and another for cows' milk. Today's there's no need to go to the Dairy Co-op, Mummy says. Today the milk is sold to Konsum.

One woman had sold enough milk to buy a new car. She had big breasts, Mummy says.

Like buckets, Daddy says. Tits as big as ten-litre buckets.

Oh, rubbish, Mummy says. But they were big.

The woman with the milk drove around in her new, shiny car with her valuable breasts resting against the steering wheel.

Four weeks had passed. It was now the children were to come home. Mummy prepared things. She rolled out a red carpet inside herself and thought out ceremonies. She walked around, more restless than ever. She washed the rooms once again. They smelled of detergent and disinfectant. The house, which had suffered and tormented itself through the winter, began slowly to recover. You can imagine how it wakes up and gradually frees itself from the foundations that hold every house firmly to the ground.

The taped windows have been freed from their strips of paper and are open wide, with the wind brushing over clean floors. The house shimmers and its spirit—yes, every house has a spirit and a soul,—its spirit flies around amongst the delicate shoots on the trees.

That was how they'd imagined it, that was why they'd bought the house. A dream-house for happy children with red cheeks and gaily coloured flowers that glow out over the surroundings.

Mummy and Daddy were summoned to the doctor at the children's hospital. He was polite. Friendly and polite, Daddy says. There was something the matter with Berit. Something to do with her lungs.

Mummy sat with her hands straight down along her sides and squeezed the edge of the chair.

We've put her in an incubator, the doctor said.

In an incubator? They stared at the doctor. The children

were supposed to come home now? They'd been promised that the children would be released now. Wasn't that why they'd been asked to come to the hospital?

She's having problems with her temperature again, the doctor said. Sometimes she changes colour.

What's wrong with her lungs? Daddy said.

We've X-rayed them and . . . the doctor paused a moment before answering. Mummy noticed the pause. By now her ears had been trained beyond their natural capacity. The pause was an avalanche that sent roof beams and boulders crashing over her.

The X-rays show shadows in her lungs, the doctor went on.

While the avalanche thundered through Mummy's head everything else in the room remained motionless.

What are the shadows due to? Daddy said.

She's already come round in the incubator, the doctor answered. Her general state is fairly good, all things considered.

All things considered! If you ignored the pictures that showed the shadows, the shadows spreading and growing in her lungs.

What are the shadows due to? Daddy asked for the second time.

We're not sure, the doctor said.

What do you think? Mummy whispered. Her voice sounded strangely mild coming from someone fighting to free herself under a world that has collapsed. Lungs can collapse. It happens suddenly and without reason in infants. Their lungs get stuck together. The tissue gets tired. Mummy talked like someone who has already grieved a while, someone who has grown accustomed to grief.

We shouldn't be too quick to draw conclusions, the doctor said. All we can do is wait and see.

Somehow or other they got out of the hospital. They didn't notice the sun and the spring, except for the fact that they couldn't see when they left the deep shadows in the entrance and, with the sun flashing in their eyes, made their way across the area in front of the entrance.

The doctor had been considerate. But he couldn't hide the fact that they were now on their way to losing one of the children. The case history says: Parents informed of uncertain situation.

Daddy started the rusty Peugeot. He'd put the basket from the twin's pram, a wide blue basket with two quilts and room for the twins to lie beside each other, in the back of the car.

They waited. Now only what was absolutely essential was done in the house. Patrick and Lisa grew quiet and helpful. I don't think Patrick stole a single moped during all that time.

Mummy entered into her sorrow. She grew incapable of interesting herself in anything. Conversation became sporadic, incoherent because the other thing was always there. The periods when she was lost, plunged in darkness, grew longer and longer, like the dark shadow that grew in Berit's lungs.

Between these periods she could notice a gradual change inside her. It's really odd, she says. There's no explaining it afterwards. You're subjected to a process, you participate in a process of getting used to it.

She was allowed to hold Berit for brief periods. She saw the colour change across Berit's body. She saw the listless gaze.

How is she doing? Mummy asked.

All things considered . . . the nurse talked the same way as the doctor. All things considered she's doing fairly well.

But. Mummy could see things were worse. She could feel it in her hands when she held Berit.

Bearing in mind the tests, the nurse went on, she's doing surprisingly well.

After a week the wearing down process was in full operation. Berit continued to get worse and Mummy was now part of the new way of looking at it.

In reality Berit was doing well. Relatively speaking. Mummy adopted the argument as her own. She almost became happy when she thought how well Berit was doing.

She said so when she came home. She repeated it for herself. The way people with cancer do. From the first tiny, innocent lump to the last stage when their bodies are clogged with tumours and their voices no longer carry. But at least they can still think. Things might be worse. Under the circumstances they're doing quite well.

After no more than two weeks they could have handed over a dead child to her. She would have stood with the child in her arms and nodded. Of course, bearing in mind the tests . . . surprising the child lasted as long as she did. All things considered, that was a favourable aspect.

A defence mechanism? Mummy says so sometimes, but she doesn't know. The mechanism wasn't faultless. Despair and insight suddenly rushed in, the periods of darkness grew longer.

I breathed and screamed. I ate and began to grow. After six weeks I was allowed to come home. They took me in through the back door. That's what it feels like when I think of it. Like when the cat carries something across the threshold.

Of course we were happy when you came home, Mummy says.

We were so busy with Berit, Daddy says.

They can't hide it. Mummy'd become desperate when I arrived. She didn't want me. After half an hour she was ill. Everything in her stomach ran out of her. Daddy wasn't at home. She was alone with me and with her feelings that chased her into areas she had never been in. She's not really like that. Her nature isn't nervous, it's never hysterical.

She's steady, Daddy says. Stubborn and steady.

I lay on the kitchen table on a light-blue blanket. Mummy walked as though in her sleep. She staggered over to the telephone. She couldn't manage any more. All she wanted to do was vomit and sit on the WC. She dialed the number to the hospital.

I can't help her, Mummy said.

What do you mean, the nurse said at the other end of the line.

I can't, it's impossible.

But really . . .

I'm ill, don't you understand? Ill!

But the girl is healthy, the nurse said.

I have a stomach ailment! Mummy sent off a series of desperate cries for help. I'll contaminate her! I can't touch her, I can't give her food!

I realize you've been under heavy pressure, the nurse said.

You must take her back, Mummy said.

That's out of the question.

I'm on my way in with her, Mummy said. I'll take the car and I'll be there in half an hour.

Unfortunately—the nurse said.

Mummy had slammed down the receiver. She wanted to give me back to the hospital. They didn't want me. No one wanted me.

You can't blame them. Everyone says that. I've heard myself say it.

They didn't want me and Berit took first place. Once I pushed her out of bed. She was in a bunk bed. She broke her arm.

I did it although I know no one is to blame. I love her. We've grown up together. She helps me. Like a close friend. She's the finest person I know.

And yet I could push her out again when I think of what happened then. Berit blocked the view. They couldn't see what they should have seen in me.

How can you say a thing like that? Granny asks.

They didn't care, I say.

They loved you so.

Not me.

Granny bends over my bed and pushes her nose against mine. We laugh. One has a right to be unfair. A need even. Children need to be unfair to provoke what they long to hear. That they're loved.

Asa's fishing, Berit says teasingly.

Granny's voice is like a pillow you lay your head against. She tells me about the birth. She has boxes and when she opens them the room falls under a spell. I think I was five when I heard her tell about it the first time. After that I wanted to hear it again and again.

She's close to what's old and fabulous. Once upon a time mankind was born from moss and heather. Man worshipped the sun and the rain. He made sacrifices to the earth and prepared himself for the sacred meeting.

What meeting? I ask although I already know.

The meeting between heaven and earth. Mankind gathered on the mountain to propitiate the gods, the rain and sun gods who gave life.

When did that happen? I whisper.

In the spring, always in the spring. I take her hand and put it against my mouth. I lie and snuffle against her hand and listen to the birth. It's my spring and my birth.

There are no case histories from the old years. Granny opens new boxes and no matter how hard you look you won't find incubators, bacteria or twisted legs. People sang and played. It sometimes happened that the women danced naked.

That's where the fairy tales begin, Granny says. And the theater.

Daddy's theater, I say?

I don't think so, Granny says.

A small laugh bubbles up somewhere inside her. Now that I'm older I understand why. Daddy wrote plays about workers. They were always dressed, they wore helmets and they took snuff. Imagine if they were naked! The factory doors open and naked workers pour out, singing a hymn to a huge spanner.

Daddy would have become angry if he'd heard Granny's laugh. As a matter of fact he was already angry. He crept up on us. He found pretexts and his face looked dark and strange.

Granny speaks about the sacred meeting. One day mankind gathered together all the gods, the rain and the sun and everything in the heavens. Of all of these, man made a single god. The Virgin Mary was the ground that had lain barren and desolate.

And then the child was born.

I was born in the spring, I say.

Granny nods.

But not Jesus? I breathe into her open hand. Jesus wasn't born in the spring.

Of course he was born in the spring, Granny says. It's obvious. Otherwise there would have been no point to the whole thing, no point at all. It was the Church that changed his date of birth. Jesus was born in the spring and died in the autumn. When the leaves fall.

Daddy prowls around angrily but he's not let into our conversations. He says that Granny uses black magic. Granny is religious. Once he shouted after her when she'd gone. He hissed something about Albania. I don't think he'd do it now, but he did it then. In Albania they know how to deal with religious people, he said. There they play basketball in the churches.

Granny gives meaning to things one can't discover on one's own.

But those who are ill, I object. If a baby is ill when it's born? Who dances and sings when the sick babies are born?

Granny's narrow face grows troubled in the shadows of the room. She's struggled with that question herself and she hasn't found any good answer.

You're not ill, Asa, she says and closes the last box. You're healthy.

§

What a wonderful time, what a wonderful summer it became! They moved from the house and the city. Against the horizon I can see Aunt Tilly flap and wave her stick as she stands there surrounded by second-hand household appliances, advantageous offers and everything that's indispensible and that you can't simply go off and leave behind.

They packed us, the children, into the car. Berit was home. After two months she was finally home. And now they rolled out into the summer, exhausted after their forced march through the valleys of death. Welcome back! Summer stood wide open with a loving embrace.

They never tire of talking about it. Daddy's put together several boxes of slides. I never grow tired of looking at them. Tell me about what it was like when I was small!

The car growled indolently out through yellow fields and past bathing lakes which are always warm. Patrick and Lisa pressed their faces against the car windows and squealed with delight. Summer is full of ice-cream. They must have stopped at every petrol station to buy more ice-cream. Mummy sat with her eyes half closed in the middle of the rear seat. With one hand she held the twins' basket behind her. She felt the heat of our bodies and she felt her anguish reluctantly drag itself off with its evil eyes.

We'd conquered death! It was a voyage of triumph.

They'd rented a cottage in Sörmland in southern Sweden. The car turned off from the asphalted road and rocked like a desert camel under its load of beds and mattresses, suitcases and bundles. It sniffed its way along narrow gravel roads with a strip of grass down along the centre. And there it was! Daddy stopped the car in a glade. Patrick and Lisa rushed out. Daddy and Mummy sat on in silence.

It was a real farm cottage. With white-painted corners, a maid's room in the loft, a pressure tank and hot-water radiators that had been connected to the heart of the house, a big wood stove. There were apple trees, berry bushes and a barn. Time had left its mark, as had the lightning that had once struck the house. The house had been knocked about. Yet, it was in fine form as it lay there in its own world with the forest encircling the small farmyard and the meadow below it.

They sat in silence with the engine switched off. They stared as though overcome by the rapture they now felt. Here was the first-aid station the wounded search for.

If only the children stay healthy, Mummy thought.

It's over now, Daddy thought.

§

They sank into each other and into the summer. Days and nights danced past like the down-white balls that danced across the meadows. Sörmland is forest, Daddy says. He walked for hours amongst elks and foxes.

Sörmland is deer, Mummy says. She and Daddy sat on the slope outside the cottage with the round glow of the paraffin lamp like a moon above the garden table. They listened to the deer call at the edge of the meadow. Night sounds are terrifying until you learn what they are. Like screams from tormented children. They were still sitting there when the morning crept in with dew and paling stars, and they saw the deer graze on the meadow.

They made love and kissed and gasped when the thunder and the rain built black towers amongst the clouds. There's no thunder like the thunder in Sörmland, Daddy says. The rain was torrential, the thunder crashed like sheets of iron above their heads. They had never heard such noisy thunder as they heard that summer. It was a warning, Daddy says. They reached out for each other. They took care of their children. They approached each other with friendly words like gifts from travellers who have been far away. One day as they sat in the kitchen and the thunder crashed above the roof and the telephone rang, a huge fireball rolled out from the stove and across the floor.

Daddy shows me a picture of the car as it stands parked with the door open. There, he says, and points with a pen under the dashboard, there a field mouse hid. It ate the electric cables. I couldn't get it out.

One day when he was driving along the motorway south of Stockholm—he was driving fast, he likes driving fast—the mouse went mad. It climbed up his trouser leg, passed his knee and on up.

Oh, Mummy says.

It was awful, Daddy says. But I managed to stop the car.

Just imagine, Mummy says and smiles happily.

They babble and make their way forward through the summer. This is their favourite memory! We carry our memories in a basket with us through life. We pick them out, we can throw them at ghosts and at the shadows of despair. We draw a circle of happiness around our little world. We do it because outside that world is the other world, the world we dread.

Bitter salt, Granny says. The best memories contain something bitter. You have to have tasted it to really be able to feel it.

Daddy took photographs. It's all there in the photos, the sweet and the bitter.

§

The night breathes and its breath is greyer now. The rabbit sits huddled up with her unchanging eyes on the window. I shiver and close the window, carefully so as not to wake those who are asleep.

The rabbit hutch stands on the lawn below the window. I can see the mat, the gym mat, that covers the hutch. The shiny, red side is facing upwards and I see it against the dark grass of the lawn.

The doctor from Prague disappears from my story. He

disappears for a while and I don't really know what he's doing. It's like when your eyes get narrower and narrower and you see flashes of fragmented pictures just before you fall asleep.

The doctor is working. That much I realize. He works feverishly night and day. Man's lifespan on earth isn't enough. The children are always there as are the waiting mothers in the queue to the clinic. The documentation, the theoretical work must be carried out again. New archives, new case histories. Everything that was lost must be built up again now that evil has rolled in over the city of Prague. The children of the world wait.

Can we catch up with our own future? Practical problems stand in the way and pile up. Like a lumberjack we must saw and break our way through the days and clear away the obstacles to reach the moment when what is significant is to be measured.

I can see him sitting, just as I sit, beside an open window and suddenly discovering how he shivers in the cold air that he'd forgotten exists. He closes the window and rubs his hands a moment to create a little warmth. If only he weren't so tired! His family is doing well. His wife, ever patient, watches understandingly as he rushes past the dining-table on his way to the clinic.

New physical therapists must be trained, routines must be created, a throng of simple and trivial problems must be solved to make the next day possible. It is not until afterwards, when everyday life has gone to bed and the lamps have been put out, that there is time for what is most important. That time must be picked out of everyday life the way the kernal is picked out of a nut.

It is then, when your eyes burn with tiredness, that your brain has to work with the greatest precision. The doctor refines his theories. The theories will determine everything. Science will never recognize his work if his theories are unclear. With their aid he'll convince those who are most difficult to convince. The words he's written dance across the paper in front of him. He must arouse new sources of strength if he is not to fall asleep.

He and those like him always have back-up batteries. Extraordinary people like him who move out in no-man's land triumph over their tiredness.

What is it that drives him? I torment myself with that question. The doctor from Prague gets comfort from the cross he carries but I'm almost certain his cross never gives him any answers to this, the most important of questions. I hear myself scream. I'm blue, blue as my legs were at the moment of birth. My scream tears down the noble motives. The doctor from Prague works himself to death but he doesn't do it for the children's sake. Don't believe that. Not in the last analysis. And not for his family's sake, the family he seldom has time to meet. Not even for his own sake.

I once read about chimpanzees. The answer to why researchers and artists take such pains can be found amongst the chimpanzees. They put a banana outside the chimpanzee's cage. They gave the chimpanzee two sticks that could be joined together. If the chimpanzee managed to join the sticks together he could reach the banana.

He failed. He worked himself into a fury and poked the sticks between the bars. He struck them against the floor in front of the banana and screamed. At last he gave up. He turned his back on the banana and began to play with the sticks instead. And then, playing, he joined the sticks together. Not until then, when the actual purpose of doing it had been forgotten and the game had taken over, did he succeed.

The truth about the pains researchers take, the furious efforts, the blind game, can be found in the chimpanzee's cage. The doctor from Prague classifies his children and plays his way forward, flogging his weary body with new tasks. He does it out of curiosity, he does it for the same reason small children put their fingers into an electric socket. Is this the truth about their expedition into my brain, their journey through my body? If only I knew!

One evening the doctor is sitting with a letter in his hand. That I know for certain. He's being asked to travel north. Others too have fled from Prague. One of his assistants, a physical therapist, has settled down in Stockholm. There they want to hear the doctor from Prague. Their interest has been aroused. He puts the letter to one side. The invitation is a sign of success. His desk is covered with photographs of children. He studies the photographs. His eyes are trained. He can see at once if there's anything unnatural about the children. He can see it even in infants, even as young as six months.

A method for investigating, a system. It's called early diagnosis. The doctor from Prague works on it tonight and for a hundred nights to come. I've spread out the photos from that first summer. Daddy mostly took slides that can be shown on the wall. But he took ordinary photos as well, enough to cover many desks. In one of the photos, a colour photo that he's had blown up, is the key to the closed doors of my story.

They've laid out a light-blue blanket on the grass. It must be outside the summer cottage. You can glimpse a few currant bushes at the edge of the photo. My sister Berit and I are lying on our stomachs on the blanket and Mummy and Daddy and the other children are round about.

Daddy must have put the camera on a stone and pressed the delayed-action release. Then he ran and threw himself down amongst them, you can see that because he only got half way down. They're all laughing and their laughter has burst out amongst the clover and the pale meadow flowers.

Berit lies with her legs pulled up under her. Her behind is sticking up and she's soft as a ball. I don't lie like that.

Asa's funny. I hear the delighted exclamations of that first summer. Asa is pretty.

I lie with my legs stretched out. My neck is bent backwards. Everything seems stretched, even my feet. My toes point inwards at an angle.

How pretty! Mummy had left her house of sorrow, she'd

pulled down the dark curtains, she'd opened wide the doors and finally gone out into the summer. Asa is pretty, she said but she kept her gaze fixed on Berit, the child who'd been so close to death. Yes, they had to keep a careful watch over Berit.

So it continued. All that summer and half the autumn.

They shared us. They almost competed about feeding us and changing us and letting us lie naked across their naked bodies in the mornings.

Berit continued to be their soft ball. Soon she was lying on her back and sucking her toes. Children do that to train their trunk muscles. They play with their toes to learn to raise their backsides. They train turning around for the first time.

I didn't suck my toes. I didn't train to turn around. They thought my stretched body was a peculiarity of mine. They saw my wandering eyes that went round and round and wouldn't stop. Infants find it difficult to fix their gaze. That's natural and after all there was nothing wrong with my eyes. The case history is reassuring about that. No sunset, it says. If you have a sunset your pupils are like setting suns at the bottom of your eyes, with the whites showing above. In that case you can get water on the brain.

My eyes whirled round like the eyes of the Negro dolls they used to have in the amusement park in Tivoli, Daddy says. When you put a coin in the dolls their eyes began to whirl round.

My eyes were turned not downwards like sunsets but upwards. You can see the whites beneath. They all sat around the blanket and saw my peculiar eyes and were happy.

Asa is such an individual, Mummy said. How different they are!

There are no brothers or sisters as different as fraternal twins, Daddy said.

They invited their friends around. The theater Rabble came rattling along the forest roads in their old bus. They came with their guitars and their songs. They gathered around our blanket and admired. Daddy gave a talk. His strength and his virility were demonstrated.

Look how different they are! The heads moved up there above me and my sister Berit. There were cheers and songs for us and for the sunset.

Everything develops contrarily in fraternal twins, Daddy said during one of his eternal lectures. In the old days they killed twins. It's against nature to give birth to more than one child, it's animal.

An actress giggled in the shadows behind a door. Someone was squeezing her breast.

Only animals are multiparous, Daddy went on. A newly-born child has God as its Godfather. But if two are born, the other Godfather must be the devil.

Nature creates opposites, Daddy said. He took out the little red book the Chinaman had written. The science of opposites is called dialectics.

He'd got hold of that mystical word—the fat Chinaman was really Mummy's department, but Daddy wasn't altogether free from his influence either and now he pressed that little word to his heart. I think the Rabble had an almost boundless admiration for him in those days—after all, most of them were scarcely literate.

Daddy unfolded the word in front of his astounded listeners. Dialectics. If one fraternal twin is carefree, the other becomes reserved. If one forgives, the other fights. The difference is there in their souls, it's not something you have control over, you can't develop it, life bounces forward between opposites.

The dialectics of twins! I can't stand that word and, as usual, I sulk when he talks about us as though we were a unit.

Look, even in appearance you can see the difference, Daddy called.

My failing eyes haven't retained a picture of the throng of people who passed by. The Rabble, their faces fuddled with wine and food, Aunt Tilly's searching birdlike gaze when she visited us. In autumn, when we were back in town, other people would come and look and see for themselves. It was like a rush-hour queue for the underground.

They saw us. And yet no one saw. Not for the first five months.

I pick up the picture and hold it close to the lamp. Now I can see it clearly. Berit has managed to get her elbows beneath herself. My arms are stretched out along my sides. If I use a magnifying glass I can study my hands. My thumbs are turned into my palms.

How pretty Asa is! Everything about that child is pretty. Even her thumbs.

I've put pressure on Mummy. I've crossed-questioned her. I've forced her to admit it. There was something she noticed. Berit opened her hands, her infant grip opened up. I didn't.

My toes are turned inwards like my thumbs.

We were so happy that summer, Mummy says.

You noticed, I say.

Your thumbs were so small, Mummy says. I couldn't imagine there were going to be any problems. Not with thumbs as small as that.

§

Daddy threw himself into a new project that autumn. He worked like a madman. He rushed in, read what he'd written out loud and rushed off again. A new boiler was installed in the house.

Mummy was going to stay at home for another few months. She gave time to Lisa and Patrick. She went through their homework with them, she busied herself with Lisa who had become almost crazy with jealousy when we were in the hospital. Lisa got a new bow in her hair and a school bag. Lisa became a big girl. The school flag was run up and the teacher bid the children welcome in her finest dress.

Things were different then, Daddy says. Growing up meant something. Now children are slipped gently into it. They're sneaked into school. They're softened up and tenderized. Their heads are filled with jelly so they don't even notice the decisive moments in their lives.

Things were better in the old days, Mummy says ironically.

Rubbish, Daddy says.

Lisa stalked off to school on her thin legs with a bag that was far too big, with a bow in her hair and great seriousness written all over her being.

Patrick had thrown stones at cars from a bridge. Mummy got hold of him, she had meetings with the school and with other parents. It turned out that Patrick had done other dreadful things. He was pointed out as the ringleader when his class threw pizzas at the domestic science teacher. Now things were going to be put to rights. Mummy was elected chairman of the parent-teacher association. Despite her green tuft and her red hair. The neighbours began to be polite to her. Her politicals swarmed into the house. They hadn't learnt to be polite yet.

The house smelt of baby food and nappies. Daddy came home to infant smells. He looked out over Mummy's chaos like a commander who regards a battlefield and has just found out that the war is over.

This place looks like hell, he said happily.

I haven't had time, Mummy said.

She's always tried to convince him that she grew up on a backyard in the centre of Stockholm. He doesn't believe her. He says she spent her first fifteen years in a boarding house. He says there's no other explanation. She's a boarding house woman.

At least it's clean, Mummy said.

Clean as hell, he said.

You might think they were having a row. You have to

know them to understand. They almost never had rows that autumn. The warmth of summer hung on and sizzled in every corner.

Aunt Tilly was allowed to come. Daddy tamed her. No one could explain how he did it. Maybe he used a whip.

You have to show her cold steel sometimes, Daddy says. There are few people who can be as nice as Aunt Tilly. As long as you wave cold steel under her nose.

It almost became the proper family Daddy dreamed of. Mummy sat obediently at the kitchen table in the late evening and listened when he read what he had written. While the little elves slept, Daddy elf told how he'd hunted the wicked snake. Soon Mummy was going to start working again. We were to be put in a day nursery. Every little nerve inside her began to send out small signals of longing. She prepared herself, although she gave herself a little longer to enjoy the role of guardian of the larder with the key in her apron.

Daddy read. She lit a candle and wondered how long you can look at the flame without blinking.

Are you listening?

Oh, yes, she said.

Isn't it good?

It's wonderful.

He read on. What he had written was a sort of assurance. There was something wrong in his theater. It had begun to boil somewhere down at the bottom. The theater was a pressure cooker.

I've laid the keel for the new play, he said. I've laid out the frame.

Don't they want it?

Maybe. I think they're preparing to revolt. Caesar is to be assassinated.

Send Aunt Tilly to them, Mummy said.

She's already there. He polished his glasses. When you get down to it, every actress is like Aunt Tilly. They'd put their own children in the oven and set it at three hundred degrees for a good part.

That's not fair, Mummy said.

Not fair to whom?

To Aunt Tilly. Why don't you write some good parts for them?

I think they're tired of workers, Daddy said. They're going around with lists.

It didn't really matter to him. He was still back there in the summer and in the feeling he had when he threw himself fearlessly off the rock into the little forest lake.

They blew out the candle. They took each other by the hand and climbed the stairs, shy as though they were fourteen years and had just met at a school dance.

They stood in the smell of babies and looked at Berit and me. Mummy had thought of asking about me. Berit was already up on her knees while I lay so strangely stretched out. Mummy had made an appointment with a doctor in town.

Asa's coming on, Daddy whispered.

§

The doctor was one of the wise and careful doctors that developments had missed. They'd gone around with smoke and noise, changing everything, but this doctor had held out in one of the labyrinthine hideaways where the smoke hadn't yet reached. His flat in the fashionable Östermalm district was old and surrounded the visitor with even older wisdom. The doctor himself made one think of crystal. He used the old, classical methods. As long as the city could remember he had cared for the city's children. As his father had before him.

Now he was troubled. He analyzed his observations and cautiously structured what he had seen. He wasn't sure, he emphasized that several times. But it seemed best to write out a referral note to a specialist, a specialist in neurology.

Mummy sat on a low, ancient chair with me on her knee. Berit crept about on the floor while the doctor's words still refused to give up their content.

Neurology? Is there something wrong with her nerves?

The doctor had devoted almost an hour to examining us. The idea of fast consultations didn't exist in his surgery. His method was surveillance, watching carefully over what determines the normal flow of life in infants.

Why had Mummy come?

For a triple vaccination, Mummy said.

The doctor fixed two all-seeing eyes on me.

The child welfare centre doesn't function very well, Mummy went on.

No? Mummy looked uneasy. Perhaps it was exaggerated to go to the leading doctor in town for a vaccination. But at the child welfare centre they said something about being understaffed and, besides, the doctors were involved in a salary dispute.

Mummy held on to us while the doctor began his examination. It was me he devoted his time to, a lot of time and a lot of methodically penetrating questions.

What does the Sachsska Children's Hospital say, the doctor asked?

Should they say something?

Haven't they asked you to come in?

No, Mummy said.

Odd. He placed me on an examination table and turned and twisted my body. He was bewildered and he didn't hide it.

Prematurely born children are usually called in for a check, he said.

But if everything is normal maybe it's not needed, Mummy said, trying her way forward with weak assumptions.

The doctor took out a little bell. He rang the bell carefully beside my ear. I didn't react. He rang it harder. There was no reaction.

Is she deaf? he asked.

No.

Are you sure of that?

Mummy nodded and felt an alien coldness burrow its way into her diaphragm. The rest was a nightmare and fear that sank like a stone through clear water.

Something with her nerves?

The doctor was busy writing out the referral note. He put down his pen and studied the perplexing observations about my body and my lack of reaction. He didn't say that but it was quite clear nevertheless and finally Mummy formulated it in a rasping voice.

So Asa's brain is damaged?

The doctor spoke with all the calm and wisdom of his experience. He used his voice as one might inject a tranquilizer in a victim crushed beneath a wrecked car. There are so many possibilities. In any case Asa must be checked by a specialist.

And if?

The doctor went on with his analysis, methodically and very cautiously. Mummy heard him as she lay there crushed in the wrecked car while the tranquilizing painkiller tried in vain to spread in her body.

It was a suspicion, he said. Perhaps there was no basis for it. As a general practitioner he refused to go into the question of treatment. Particularly since treatment might not be needed at all.

Is there any cure?

The doctor stroked his iron-grey hair. He'd used up his store of lifebelts and tranquilizers. He balanced on the very limit of caution when he spoke about the new method.

A doctor from Prague has developed a method for training brain-damaged children.

Is it effective?

It's highly disputed. I don't know any more than that, the doctor said and handed over the referral note to Mummy. She left the doctor's surgery. So far, what he had said contained nothing but an ill-fated conclusion. She eased the pram over the threshold and into the treacherous ground that lay ahead.

She pushed her little ones in front of her. She and they, everyone in the little family, had made their way out of the gloomy days that followed the delivery. It was like walking without noticing that you're walking on a belt moving in the opposite direction. When you look around again you're back in the world of case histories and monstrous fear.

The suspicions in the referral note were concentrated unhappiness. It was a misty November day and the mist washed against her face. The street sang a hostile song with shrill engine noises and whining tyres, a battlesong, and with it came vague ideas of the mishapen, the wretched one observes briefly before tactfully looking away.

She had been on the move. One summer morning she'd boarded a train with her family, a train loaded with flowers and comforting words. A train of happiness, a train for safe travel, a train in which you can fall asleep while the days and hours thump by along the rails. But someone was moving about while they slept. Someone switched the points and when she woke up the train had come to a standstill in a swamp and the future waited out there with its poisonous breath.

Already, as she pushed her pram and her world before her, the hunt had started inside, the murderous hunt for guilt, the guilt she would torment herself and those around her with. Of course there were gaps in the first reports from the doctors, but the important gaps didn't concern the bacteria in Berit's lungs, the gaps she'd thought she'd detected and uncovered. Their only purpose was to hide the other gaps, the important gaps. She'd been the victim of a trick, a double trick.

Why hadn't they informed her about the risks of premature birth? Why hadn't she learnt to see? Every little detail in the behaviour of my stretched-out body, everything that had seemed so amusing and individual now emerged as a confirmation of unforgivable blindness.

Why had they been pushed out of the hospital without being called in for a subsequent check-up? All hospitals check up on premature births. All proper hospitals.

We should have tried to have you moved. Aunt Tilly reminded her later.

It wouldn't have worked, Daddy said. There's no point in rummaging around in all that.

Aunt Tilly wouldn't give up. She only said what everyone knew. Everyone who had been born and who had their roots in the cracks between the city's stones. It was a pauper's hospital! With medical students and trainee doctors who rush around and end up not knowing their own names, much less those of the patients. Who train on ordinary people before they open their own practice or take up a position in the shade of the balconies of the houses of the rich.

To say nothing of the surgical department!

Stop, Daddy said. We can't take any more of that just now.

In the surgical department the chief surgeons fight with each other, Aunt Tilly ground on. It was even in the papers. Fist fights. They countermand each other's prescriptions.

Daddy literally carried Aunt Tilly out. Out of hearing range of Mummy. Now there were new suspicions to measure. Guilt! Young women smoke and drink wine.

Daddy got furious. Mummy had scarcely touched a glass of wine since she became pregnant.

But she smokes. Aunt Tilly muttered behind Mummy's back. And what about the abortion. Didn't Mummy have an abortion once? An abortion tears apart a woman's insides. That's why so many children are born too early and are damaged. It's unnatural to have abortions. We live in an unnatural age. Abortion on demand! Aunt Tilly was a witch who held her last, dark sermon before being burned at the stake. There's a price to pay. The children have to pay it for women's lust and convenience!

§

Mummy pushed the blue pram through the city. She stopped, bent down and adjusted our quilts. We slept deep inside the primeval dreams of children, untroubled by the hostility of the street. Mummy continued under the Christmas lights. The shopkeepers had installed them like a vault across the streets in a joint effort to sell Christmas cheer on credit well in advance.

She wasn't looking where she was going. She was pushed and she staggered out onto the street. A driver wound down his window and shouted things about her sex after her. City people puff around with hysteria as their last fuel. Their nerves are burnt and leave a smell of singed fibres behind them.

An old-age pensioner stood in front of the pram. He gave out because Mummy, in a new and clumsy move, had run the pram over his foot. Of all the people in the city the pensioners are the worst. Daddy usually says that. They push their way to the front of the queues, they shout their way forward, they don't like prams on buses, they shoplift and they hate young people.

Mummy neither heard nor saw when the city growled and snapped its teeth after her. A taxi! She clung to the idea that a taxi would be her salvation. She managed to stop one. She sank into the seat, weighed down by guilt and new questions. Her fault? Had she led a careless life? Was she the cause of it all?

She pressed her children against her. I stretched my neck backwards. She felt my tense body and added new explanations to old observations. My tongue! I pushed out the comforter with my tongue.

She picked up the comforter, which had fallen on her knee. Defective children have difficulty talking, they can't control their tongues. For the last few months she'd been wondering about the fact that I pushed food out with the tip of my tongue. My tongue was pushed forward in my mouth, I had difficulty eating and difficulty holding on to the comforter and difficulty keeping food in my mouth.

Where to? the driver said.

What? Mummy said.

What address?

Rosenvägen, she muttered.

Where's that?

Drive south.

The driver turned around and looked at her with his brow furrowed. Wasn't she feeling well, could he help with anything?

When the taxi arrived at our house Daddy was home. The driver put the pram on the pavement. Mummy left it there. She kept us pressed against her body. She hadn't changed her grip since she got into the car. She crossed the threshold. It was first then that she began to cry. Her tears were a flood that swept the last of her consciousness away. She told them straight out. Asa has cerebral palsy!

§

I pull down the theater in front of me on the desk. I change the story to a film. I see Mummy sink into the sofa and Daddy bend over her.

It's like a film. I cut and insert the doctor from Prague and adjust the focus. He arrives at Stockholm. He's received with love and consideration. He meets his former assistant, the physical therapist from Prague. They were in Yugoslavia at the same time when Prague was invaded. They fled the country at the same time. He embraces her.

Flight makes brothers and sisters of people. So much to be said and so many new things to recount. Our successes in Cologne are unquestionable, he says. Now Stockholm is on its way to being won. A clinic has been opened on St. Paulsgatan.

Journalists are waiting at the airport when he arrives. The newspapers say that there's a glimmer of hope for defective children. The doctor from Prague is presented as a miracleworker who can cure spastic children and get the lame to walk.

People really want to listen to him. The lecture hall is packed. A lot of them are enthusiastic. He begins his lecture by saying a few words about the newspapers. He can't cure spastic children. He can't do it and nor can anyone else.

He sees the audience smile. Newspapers shouldn't be taken too seriously. They create headlines.

He speaks to the doctors in the lecture hall, particularly to the neurologists. As they know, damage caused by cerebral palsy can't be cured, the brain is and remains damaged. On the other hand . . . he looks out over his audience and notes a reaction he can't interpret. On the other hand, it is possible to break through the blocks.

Someone bends forward and whispers to him. He's been talking to non-existent listeners. There are no doctors in the lecture hall, none of the important doctors. At that moment the doctor from Prague realizes that his journey has been a failure.

He completes his lecture. But he knows that he's failed. They haven't taken the trouble to come and listen, the strategists, the brain specialists. Of course those who are present listen but that's not enough. They absorb his lecture as though he were serving them a life-giving drink. He builds up his theoretical structure in front of their hopeful eyes and at the same time he longs to return to the security of his own clinic in Cologne.

At the end of the day they crowd around him to thank him. He forces out a smile and takes leave of them as though they were all about to go on board a plan he knows will crash. In the middle of this tumult he's attacked by a furious woman. He's a charlatan, doesn't he know that? He has no scientific evidence! Her words are coarse and are deformed by her poor mastery of German. The doctor's method is cruel, it destroys the children. Torture! She holds onto his arm and her fingers dig in like claws. She talks the way someone who hates talks.

The doctor from Prague looks around. Her claws have released their grip and the woman has disappeared. In the general confusion nobody but he noticed the attack. The arrangers present him with flowers. They are women who, with their own hands, have sought out the forgotten children and, with those same hands, have tried to master relentless nature, nature which twisted the children like pieces of crooked wire.

You should have invited the doctors, he says, exhausted after a day of complete concentration.

We did invite them.

Why didn't they come?

No one knows for sure. A mistake had been made. The whole thing should have been arranged through the Medical Society. Doctors should preferably be invited by doctors. Sergeants don't change generals' maps and corporals don't start a war without asking their captains. But it wasn't really as bad as all that . . . was it?

The doctor from Prague holds the flowers in front of his face. He hides his face in the flowers they've given him. The scent of innocence! What would the world look like without the innocent?

PART TWO

Chapter Seven

They gathered in front of the door leading out to the unknown. They prepared their expedition, they wrote lists of equipment and made an effort to talk about practical details to avoid thinking too much about what was out there.

Their voices reach me clearly now while the house and the city are rocked by the slow pulse of existence at rest. The only ones not asleep are those whose hearts are about to break.

I too am awake. I am a solitary pilot guiding my plane between the continents. Fifteen thousand metres above the ground, alone with the blue dashboard lights, I fly like the last survivor, the last witness who saw the Milky Way go out.

My story longs to rest. I take the rabbit and put her on my knee. She trembles and scrapes a little with her claws. When Daddy was small Aunt Tilly rented a cottage. That was during the war. Aunt Tilly bought a hutch with rabbits.

Daddy loved the rabbits. He gave them names. He fed them and played with them. Towards the end of the summer they disappeared, one by one. Pelle and Olle and all the rest. Daddy cried. It was probably the fox, Aunt Tilly said. The fox is the most cunning animal of all.

But it wasn't the fox. It was Aunt Tilly. When Daddy was asleep she slaughtered the rabbits. They were short of food. She earned so little. She minced their meat and mixed it with fish. Out of consideration for Daddy she didn't want to serve the rabbits the way they were.

Daddy ate meatballs made of the rabbits and didn't know he had just eaten up little Pelle who had such a sensitive nose. He thought they were fishballs. Towards the end of the summer he became ill with worry. He couldn't sleep. He kept watch over the rabbit hutch with the last rabbit. But he couldn't keep it up. Sleep took hold of him and when he woke the last rabbit was gone.

I should rest, I and my story. But if I fall asleep they'll take hold of my story. They'll kill it. Ever so kindly, ever so considerately they'll clean out my story and mince it in the we-understand-exactly-how-you-feel mincer. Then I'll have to eat it up. They'll serve it for dinner the way Aunt Tilly served the rabbits. Then my story'll be fair, sensible and dead.

Asa's making it up, they'd say.

Not at all.

We have a better memory of it than you.

I have to do it this way.

Why?

Because I have to.

I hear their voices. I was eight months old and they were talking about the expedition they'd planned. When Lisa had been tucked in and Patrick had been examined on his homework they spoke with low voices and with the intensity of those who know that silence is their enemy. Silence contains what we don't know. And can't know. They talked themselves to sleep and then they talked themselves awake.

Their words were like a spell to ward off their own uncertainty. I can scarcely imagine being worse prepared for carrying out the task they had now decided to carry out.

I'd call them weak, victims, blown hither and thither. I know that Daddy can rattle on threateningly with his typewriter and that Mummy can sound like a successful lawyer when she begins to discuss business. But that's not what

I'm talking about. I'm talking about what existed between the walls in our home. That inside world. I'm talking about Daddy who almost broke down at the slightest shift in tone. Daddy, who hurt so many and made fun of so many people in his plays, wears his own nerves like a knitted pullover around his body.

And Mummy who is so contradictory in what she says and does about things at home that she can seldom give a straight yes or no when you ask her something. For safety's sake she answers both yes and no. At the same time.

Daddy says that it's got worse with the years. She wasn't like that then. He says she should stop using Mum under arms. She should stop cooking in aluminium pots. You end up with lumps of aluminium in your head. He's bought pills with selenium for her. They'll help, he says.

I don't care what they say. That's part of their eternal war. I know what they're like in their hearts. They're as uneasy as steam above a boiling pot. They're weak now and they were weak then.

Supported against each other they stood in front of the door leading out into the unknown. I lay in front of them. The door they opened was me.

They were going to conquer the universe. That was the crazy ambition they had as they made their way out into the unknown. The universe means the divine order. I know. You can look up words like that. But God wasn't too successful when it came to creating order. Maybe He doesn't even exist. They were going to do what God couldn't do. Put the landscape in order, the landscape where the nerve systems lay like dried-out riverbeds in my brain.

They thought everything was possible. It was only a matter of wanting enough. Infinity is a circle, you reach out and take hold of it, you burn your fingers but if you make an effort you can almost force it apart, straighten it out. Mummy read about the God Thor who wrestled with the old woman who was old age. He wrestled with her and almost got her down. Almost.

They were on their way. The number of cells in the brain is like the number of stars in the skies. You can't imagine the number. Daddy made a drawing. He took it from some scientific book. Ten raised to the power of ten it says. If you count the number of brain cells at the rate of one cell a second and you do it night and day it would take you about four hundred years. Each brain cell has between a thousand and a million connections with other cells. And in several different ways. If you placed all the small nerve fibres in the brain one after another they'd reach to the moon.

They opened the door. I can imagine their reaction. How they first stood there, transfixed, with their rucksacks, their equipment and their ambitions, their helplessness which is not part of this world but of the other world, out there in what is unimaginable. The connections between the stars had broken down. The Milky Way was extinguished.

§

They were on their way. But one document was still missing, the passport they needed, the safe-conduct out into what no one has seen and no one knows anything about.

It's called a referral note. The old pediatrician had written one out. They needed another. You have to have a referral note to get a referral note.

One day in November they travelled all the way into the hospital in Kungsholmen in Stockholm. A new children's hospital with the same fluorescent tubes as in the old hospital but with more distrust smouldering in the walls. They weren't going to let themselves be pushed around. Not this time. Daddy held me in his big hands and went first through the entrance doors, his glasses misting over in the late autumn air.

They arrived with their ideas about a doctor from Prague

and about the Method that made cripples walk. They'd snapped up a few things and made a few telephone calls. The Method. The very word had a magic significance. There, where the stars had gone out, someone was prepared to show the way, to light it up with a torch.

They concealed their desperation and walked in, holding their hope in front of them like a shield.

You need to believe. That's what Granny says. You must believe in something. Those who don't believe aren't human.

The new hospital swallowed them with its orgy of rattling instruments, steel trays and a mobile sculpture in the entrance whose endless movement is supposed to put people in good humour. The doctor was a big, happy, noisy man with grey hair. He had shining teeth, sweeping gestures and a French name.

Daddy had made a preliminary investigation. That's what he calls it. There were a lot of rumours attached to the doctor's name. He had married into money and with the money he travelled all over the world representing his country. He'd almost become word famous without being invited. That's what his enemies said. But not everyone was his enemy. The doctor had also become famous for taking the children's side.

Now he stood in the deathly pale light of the children's rehabilitation clinic and held me by one of my thin legs. He made a movement downwards. He pretended to let me fall against the table.

Normal children have instincts. They resist. I didn't resist. I was cleared to zero. I didn't react to bells and I didn't resist.

Mummy and Daddy sat on their chairs. They saw the doctor test me and listened to his happy chatter. A small, powerfully built physical therapist—she looked like a fire hydrant—helped him.

What do you think? Daddy asked.

The doctor didn't answer. He went on testing. And while

he worked he filled the room with joking conjectures. Didn't they have relatives in common?

Mummy didn't think so. My body looked bluer now. But that was probably the lighting.

Or maybe they had acquaintances in common, the doctor wondered. If they talked about it a while, and he did, they'd find out that he had a sister who worked at Lisa's day nursery.

Is something wrong? Daddy said and leaned forward towards the examination table.

I'd begun to whimper. Daddy stared at the doctor's hands, his forehead wrinkled with distrust. He looked like a dog, a dog watching over a bone. What sort of an examination was this? The doctor talked nonsense and his hands seemed to work without precision. There was something indeterminate about his posture. He was chatting the way people try to chat themselves out of something awkward.

Does she react normally? Mummy asked.

The doctor lowered my naked body towards the top of the table. There are certain deviations, he said. But that isn't necessarily serious.

No?

It's difficult to say exactly. The doctor poked at me with his index finger. I lay on my stomach like a bird with my arms like folded wings along my sides.

The doctor showed his gleaming teeth. I don't think there's any need to worry.

The way she's lying, Mummy said. She got up and took me in her arms to warm me and console me.

She's just a little retarded, the doctor said.

She can't do anything, Daddy said. She can't sit, she can't turn. Nothing.

For one paralysing second he'd sunk down into the helplessness which is regarded as a pre-condition for normal intercourse between doctor and patient. Now he took hold of the conversation, he took it by the throat. They'd come here with a referral note in order to get a new referral note.

This was their chance, their only chance. They'd heard about the doctor from Prague.

I see, the doctor said.

We want a referral note to the physical therapy department, Mummy said. We want Asa to be trained according to the Method.

Once she's made up her mind she can say things unhesitatingly. Everyone realizes that discussion is superfluous. Now she sounded threatening. As though she were ready to lock the doctor into the sluicing room and keep him there as a hostage.

She said it and it was as though the lamps had gone out and the blinds had been pulled down in front of the windows. They went on talking and the doctor sounded more friendly than he had before. That's the way things work in the adult world. People pretend they don't notice.

The doctor talked a while about diagnosis. Of course he knew of the doctor from Prague. The fact of the matter was that I, Asa, had just been tested according to his system, the seven positional reflexes.

But as far as the Method was concerned . . .

What?

Actually we've tried to evaluate the Method for training physically handicapped children, the doctor said. But we've been unsuccessful.

Why?

Because you can't compare. You need a lot of children. You need material for comparisons. No one has succeeded.

So Asa is normal, Mummy said.

I haven't said that, the doctor protested.

Well, what have you said? Daddy asked.

She *may* be normal, the doctor said.

Is it because you don't want us to worry? Mummy said.

The doctor wasn't smiling any longer. The skin in his face fell down like heavy curtains over his gleaming teeth. He turned and walked out of the room.

Just a moment, he said.

They had time to get an uncertain glimpse of a tormented face before the door was sucked shut behind him. Uncomprehendingly they stared at the door and then at each other. The fire hydrant at the examination table moved. She turned a stern face towards them.

Oh, Daddy thought. He's not likely to forget that moment. Oh, we've gone too far, we've made them angry.

The physical therapist took a few steps towards them. She bent forwards and said six words, emphasizing each syllable.

You are entitled to demand it.

Then she too was gone through the door that sucked shut, sucked out and vanished in the clinking steel innards of the hospital.

What they didn't know was that the famous doctor with the French name had just left them to permit the conflict that raged inside him to sort itself out. He had, in fact, been one of the few who had introduced the Method. Now it was controversial. He himself didn't want to be controversial. He wanted to be happy and popular.

The Method meant torturing infants. There were people who claimed that. He didn't want to become known as a doctor who tortured infants. I can see myself. I can see how, naked, I stretch my over-tensed body in Mummy's arms. With an absurd logic I can't explain I'm together with the doubting pediatrician. Don't give it to them, don't give them the referral note, I beg him. Don't hand me over to them.

To understand my story you must understand how my tiny body gathered itself to resist, both then and during the years to come. How my body complained. Now, telling the story, I fill those cries of distress with words. Don't give them the referral note. My parents are fanatics. They read little red books. They get ideas. Something takes root in their heads and then off they go to the outlands of fanaticism.

Aunt Tilly laments over them. The way they live. And

they way they vote! Proper people vote for the right, she says. That's the way it's always been. But don't think your parents do. Not when they bought a house. Not even when Daddy got a grant. He got thirty thousand kroner, his name was in the papers and he was almost rich. Not even then!

They continued to vote for obscure parties that meet in attics and condemned houses. That's what Aunt Tilly says. She herself votes for the Social Democrats, I think. She votes according to her station in life. It was Mummy who got Daddy to become an extremist. After all, Daddy's almost Aunt Tilly's son. He can't have become an extremist by himself.

I see my body twist in Mummy's arms. My body is with her but there's no connection between us. I don't reach her and I don't reach the brooding doctor. My prayer remains unheard.

§

Mummy looked around the examination room and became aware of the appliances. She saw a wheelchair, a gym mat, sticks and two long bars. Some spastics can walk supported by the bars.

What would things be like for Asa? She patted me.

Asa'll become odd, ugly, mad, stupid or, in any case, unaesthetic. That was what it said in the medical encyclopaedia she'd read. Spastics look unattractive, and not only when they eat. They often drool.

Is it you they're talking about, Asa? My child!

They move with snake-like movements. That's what it said. They become like snakes.

Dear Asa! She kissed me on the forehead.

Daddy sat with his hands on his knees and squeezed them as though he could squeeze out something understandable from what had just happened. Why didn't the doctor want to write a referral note? Maybe, when you thought about it, they'd egged each other on and been swept away by a nightmare fantasy.

Maybe I, Asa, was more or less normal. Normal enough.

Mummy's green tuft wagged when she turned her head to regard the door. Her tuft wasn't funny and artistic anymore. I've read about tufts. Savage tribes paint themselves and decorate themselves with tufts. I've read about the Papuans. The Papuans look like punks. They're aggressive.

Mummy's green tuft was a declaration of war. In a world of strangers it was her way of marking her tribal affiliation. Now she was on her way out into an extinguished Milky Way. She didn't arrive as a mediator. The green tuft was her signal in the war of the stars she had just started.

The doctor sailed in through the door and the physical therapist whirled about in the current of air after him. They acted as though they'd just had a row or a fight out in the corridors.

The physical therapist rounded the doctor and the examination table. She took me out of Mummy's arms without asking. Or rather, she tore me out of Mummy's arms, she held me over the table, she made a few sudden movements from the programme the doctor had just gone through and she tried a couple of the seven positional reflexes.

Surely you can see, doctor, she said. The child doesn't react, she doesn't react at all.

It must have been an important moment for her. Several violin strings snapped in the silence that followed. When the doctor finally talked his voice was strained. Daddy claims he sounded as though he had a stick stuck up his behind.

A referral note then.

The doctor wrote. And at once they were out of his vicinity as though they were afraid he'd change his mind and take back the piece of paper. They stood outside the entrance and looked at a football pitch that lay waiting for the first winter snow.

The doctor with the French name had his revenge. He

must have regarded it as taking his revenge or as some sort of way of avoiding responsibility for himself.

In the case history in front of me on the desk he's written: Parents appear interested in physical therapy. Consequently, this was started.

As though Mummy and Daddy had some sort of perverse interest in physical therapy!

All in all, it was a good-natured revenge. It must have appeared like a brainwave later in the day when his friendly and chatty soul came into its own again. He wasn't all that cowardly, not as cowardly as he was said to be.

They got their passport with its stamp and the last, essential visa for their journey.

Send back the tickets, cancel the trip, stay at home! If my body's terror could have been expressed in words then these would have been the words to express it. I'm the solitary pilot in the night. I close my eyes and listen to my desperation. It's absurd. I have two loving and considerate parents. Despite everything I've said and everything I'm going to say, that's the truth.

I don't have to be afraid. Not for them and not for my story. I open my eyes and look out from the pilot's seat. I'll try to see what they thought they saw. The Milky Way has gone out. A cosmic sector is eliminated but not everything is dead. You can sense that if you stare at the same point for a while. You see traces, storms of energy, whirlwinds of glowing remnants that still haven't solidified.

§

They poke about in the glowing remnants. I'm lying on a new examination table. Or else it's a bed with steel tubes and green plastic covering the mattress. I'm not sure.

This is the centre, the strategists' map table. It's now they begin to sense the movement. They think they can see. They think they can hear. Everything that appeared to be dead isn't necessarily the ruins of a forgotten desert city.

My brain lives. The remnants of energy can be mobilized and new fields of force can be put to use.

They're located at the point where the two lines in my story cross. There's no need to believe in telepathy to perceive the doctor from Prague and his presence in this room. He walked in front of them with the lantern, he bent down towards ground that was lifeless and let the sand run between his fingers. Feel the warmth, the sand is warm.

Everyone who has any sense will object here. The doctor from Prague was in Germany at the time. He'd just been offered a new post and a larger clinic in Munich. He was probably sitting in a train fifteen hundred kilometres away.

And yet. A tiny particle, called an electron, can be in two places at the same time. That was demonstrated about fifty years ago. So why shouldn't a doctor be able to do it. I've followed his flight and shared his hardships. I've had him as a guest at my table. I've talked to him. This happened long before I worked up the courage to begin my story. Now he's present in a room in St. Paulsgatan in Stockholm. His world, his law! I lay on the green plastic. I was the first one to perceive the doctor's presence.

I began to scream.

It was at Christmas. When Mummy and Daddy left our house that morning the Christmas stars were alight in every window in the district. It goes against the grain to leave a warm and cozy home. They'd waited several weeks for this day. And waiting can also feel cozy and give a sort of security you get used to.

They carried me out through the front door. It was like getting up out of bed and walking straight into a cold shower. I don't know who kept an eye on Berit for them. She was already crawling around and she was always trying to turn over bookcases and throw herself down the stairs.

They waved goodbye to the children who pressed their noses against the window where the Christmas star hung. Take care of yourselves. We shan't be long.

On their way towards the trial which would strain their courage and endurance to the utmost. They'd spent the period of waiting counting days, but also with things that form part of the rituals of darkness.

They'll never abandon the Christmas star. Daddy hung it up in the window. Mummy went down to the basement with Lisa and Patrick and dug out the crêche. It's Mummy's crêche. She's had it since she was a child.

Lisa bought grass seeds and Patrick laid out soil. The shepherds and the sheep were there, as well as the wise men and the child in his little box in the crêche. Patrick put a helicopter on the crêche roof and he put a toy car amongst the shepherds outside. A sports car, Daddy claims, a Porsche. So that Joseph and Mary would be able to get away quickly when Herod thundered out against the children of Israel.

You can play endlessly with the crêche. It's always there, in the centre of every memory of Christmas, with smells of gingerbread biscuits and lighted candles round about.

Daddy bought a chime of bells with four small candles. You light the candles and fat angels swirl around amongst the delicate bells. It was a fearsome contraption and I think he put it there to make fun of Mummy's crêche.

Mummy's politicals came several times. These meetings weren't abandoned either. Mummy kept them going. She held some sort of basic course in politics. While she counted the days until everything would be as usual. As though commonplace things provided protection.

Daddy began to grow accustomed to Mummy's politicals. He called them his little Chimamen and Chinawomen, and he learned to drink tea. They talked about the poor of the world. While the fat angels swirled madly around, they talked about the Struggle.

They wondered, Mummy says. Of course they were disapproving.

But there was no trouble. Not like later when she tried to get the teachers at the day nursery to make a crêche with the children. A crêche? Never! the teachers said. There was a limit. A limit for everything.

While the days crept by, past St. Lucia with lists of presents and childish expectations of Christmas, they tried to recapture something of the playfulness of summer. People imitate the external rituals in an effort to create the internal spirit.

Mummy thought of starting work again with her clothes and the shop. As soon as they had passed the date of the appointment. As soon as they found out what was going to become of me. Daddy was having more and more trouble at the theater. Those who were critical became more numerous. But he didn't hear the criticism, he didn't see the secret alliances that were formed against him.

He saw me, the cramp in my neck and the tension in my arched body. He refused to let the trouble at the theater enter his heart and he never took it home with him. Besides, he'd had five successes in a row. He was certain that his new play would also be a success. His biggest success!

He didn't see the approaching disaster and that was my fault.

It's not true, he says. You mustn't even begin to think such a thing again. Promise me.

They left our house and its fragile idyll. Daddy drove. Mummy sat with me in the back. They looked silently out over the morning traffic and the solitary motorists who struggled against panic in the dawning civilization. They saw frost on the quays and the city, its feet washed by the deep Baltic bays.

The underground labyrinths of the Slussen clover-leaf coughed them up onto Hornsgatan. The car rounded Mariatorget. A few old men sat frozen fast on a railing. The sky lightened. The day would be clear and beautiful. Daddy drove into St. Paulsgatan and pulled up beside a parking meter.

They stood outside the door with me in a red quilted travelling bag. Mummy reached out to push the button.

She stopped the movement and let her arm drop slowly along her side. Centre for Physically Disabled Children, it said on a shining plate.

It was as though a new insight had struck her. The plate held a message that was final and offered no chance of escape. They were pigeonholed. Where they belonged, where I belonged had been decided for once and for all.

Let's not go in, she said.

What?

We don't belong here!

Daddy held me by one arm and tried to get in position to reach the button on the entrance telephone. Mummy stood in front of it.

We have an appointment, he said. They're expecting us.

I don't want to, she said.

She looked like someone talking in her sleep. He checked his watch. They still had ten minutes. With his free arm he led her out onto the street. They walked towards the bridge across the Söderleden thoroughfare. The street lamps had gone out and the cars flowed forward in a grey current beneath their feet.

She leaned against the railing. During these last days of waiting she had seen, she thought she'd seen all the broken children the city contains. She'd got new eyes and with those she became aware of the endless row of wheelchairs, tiny beings with their thumbs bent inwards, their necks angled, their legs crooked . . . She shivered and leaned further out over the railing.

Daddy held her with his hand on her shoulder. She was a sleepwalker who might well jump down into the smoking, infernal flow beneath them.

Come on, it's time, he said.

What is it that gives a human being a value? she said.

Everyone has a value. He leaned down towards her, urging her, helping her.

No value at all, she muttered.

Her eyes had looked into the forbidden city and given

her knowledge of the unspeakable. Mothers drag their mishapen children through the years, they do it for a while, a few of them manage to do it all their lives, carrying, dragging, changing nappies and feeding. But then? The wretches disappear, shovelled into the coal cellar of existence, forgotten even by the sun. Worthless!

Enormous efforts are being made for spastics, Daddy objected. There are all sorts of aids, transportation services and . . .

She turned towards him, suddenly furious at his answers. He was talking like a politician and he was lying like a politician. She hated those tactical answers. Didn't he know what every kid in every school playground knows, every kid who shouts out: Spastic!—meaning the worst scum that's every been born.

She spat the words in his face. Must one be healthy to have a value? What is it that gives Asa a value?

Her words struck him like a shower of arrows. He made no attempt to protect himself. He looked at her with the concentration of someone making a decision of vital importance.

It's us, he said. It's we who give Asa her value, you and I, no one else. That's why we're going in now. Otherwise we'll miss our appointment.

§

I lay on the green plastic, naked and wrinkled. According to the case records I weighed seven thousand, five hundred and forty-three grammes. Around me and above my head the strategists discussed me, not the doctor from Prague, not he himself since he was on his way to Munich. But the lamps in the ceiling were his eyes and the hands that worked with my body and touched the remnants of what seemed to be dead in my brain belonged to his shadow.

From here on it's the shadow that takes the doctor's place

in my story. The physical therapist. God, how I came to detest her.

She was the assistant who had fled at the same time as the doctor when Prague became dead and cold. Those who flee are dispersed by their flight. They're thrown out from the centre, they or what's left of them, they're thrown out over the world.

The doctor's shadow was square. Shadows can be square just like human beings. In any case the physical therapist made a foursquare impression. Mummy says so. Maybe it was because of fleeing and of the need constantly to build new shelters. The physical therapist seemed to be a straight sort with her character built up of right angles.

She was very resolute.

All the signs of my body were joined under her probing hands to form a picture, a picture of an illness. She worked intensively and with the searching eyes of those whose job it is to trace the innermost secrets of organisms.

They needed someone who was resolute. Daddy began to ask questions. He always wants to know everything. He got answers, but they were abrupt as the answers from an old recluse.

He said he wanted a manageable picture, a picture he could understand and work on.

Don't ask so many questions, the physical therapist said and let her hands wander on over my body, looking for new defects.

Mummy leaned down over the green cot and stroked my head. I had a pointed head then, almost like an egg. I screamed.

My scream made them uneasy. Even then I screamed with unusual savagery. And yet my scream was the scream of an infant. I've heard newly born babies scream and they sound like kittens.

Daddy regarded the physical therapist submissively. Sometimes he needs someone who puts their foot down. Who has the courage to do it. It inspires confidence.

At any rate they weren't in a position to get the entire picture clear that time, not in the state of unrelieved expectation they'd been in for so long. But they got a picture of sorts.

Daddy's put the bits and pieces together and interviewed people. It's all there in his files. If the night is long enough I'm going to read them as they're written. If the night is long enough and if you can manage to listen to the end.

That time in the room on St. Paulsgatan, at the crossroads out towards the Milky Way, they heard about athetosis. You can't expect them to have understood the word then. I still don't understand it. I was athetotic. Tonic spasms, it says in the documents. It was connected with muscle tension and relaxation. My changes were in spasms.

She's very slack, the physical therapist said. But when she stretches she tenses her muscles enormously.

There was brain damage. So much they understood. I was controlled by primitive reflexes, the reflexes which normally begin to let go when children are a few months old. I was occupied by reflexes.

While the winter morning light drifted in towards the examination room windows the strategists discussed me. I was the soldier lying on the battlefield in front of them. It was I who would win the war for them.

Is it bad? Mummy asked. She held me closer to her, her arms around my grumbling, sobbing body.

Probably, the physical therapist said.

You're not sure? Daddy asked quickly.

The physical therapist smiled a smile that was difficult to understand. Of course she was sure. But in the work she was there to do, uncertainty was an ever-present factor.

We must make more observations, she said. Then we'll see more clearly.

Mummy got up with me in her arms. Can one . . . She fumbled after what must be said, the fateful question. Can Asa become healthy?

We'll work with her, the physical therapist said. But it's already late.

She's only eight months, Mummy said.

She'll soon be nine, the physical therapist said.

She was born six weeks too early, Mummy said. Surely those six weeks should be subtracted?

Maybe. But it was fairly late. The training must begin early, preferably at six months.

Asa'll become healthy, Mummy said and pressed my head against her throat.

I was put back down in the cot. I screamed.

The physical therapist showed them. I lay on my side with my head bent forwards, one arm stretched upwards and in my hand I held the little red stick my rabbit is sniffing at in front of me now. Daddy's taken photos, I can see how I lay then. One leg was bent and fixed, my foot wasn't allowed to stretch out.

That was how I was to be trained.

I was placed in a sort of creeping position. I know how it felt. Everything seemed to be fixed in position, every part of me felt as though I were nailed to the cot. Except a single limb, my free leg that I stretched out at an angle, that I couldn't bend, that refused to allow itself to be bent.

I think I know how it felt because I screamed in such a heart-rending way, a new scream that wasn't like the earlier screams.

Mummy grew worried.

Is it painful?

No, the physical therapist said.

Then why is she screaming like that?

The Method is provocative.

Asa's a fighter. That's Daddy's way of expressing it. Screaming and spitting I was to be born again, I was to be provoked into doing it. I was right to scream, it was a good sign, he believed. But in reality, he knew almost nothing about what they were doing with me. Not then. When he tried to explain it all to himself it wasn't the language of the stars he chose but the language of the cables, electric cables.

A bit of my brain was out of function. You can run wiring in the brain just the way you can run wiring when the ignition wire in the car is burnt out, he claimed. New parts of the brain are put to use. As long as a small child's brain is still growing new paths can be created.

They were going to train me four times a day. That was what the physical therapist said they had to do. Half an hour each time. Four times a day for at least a year.

They stared dumbfounded, first at the physical therapist and then at each other. Now the full import of the plate outside the door was clear to them. Devote your life to this. Neither more nor less. You're pigeonholed.

She'll become a star gymnast, Daddy said. We'll enter Asa for the Hammarby Gymnastic Team.

I wasn't entered. Instead, I was declared a pensioner after no more than a few months. Daddy says that I got a letter and a membership card from the Swedish Pensioners' National Association. They wanted me to join them on excursions to Åland.

Don't believe him, Mummy says.

When they left the examination room they were redeemed. They thought they could see the system the doctor from Prague had conceived. They were converted to believers in a man they'd only heard rumours about. They'd met one of his disciples and immediately become members of the congregation of the faithful.

They stood in the hall in the Centre for Physically Disabled Children. I was put back in the travelling bag of red corduroy. Mummy looked around. She woke up from a confusing dream. She heard happy voices. She saw children in wheelchairs. She saw a boy who seemed to have paralyzed legs.

Children laughed. Those who were able to crept around

and played. A few parents were there, talking with soft, warm voices. They waved to her.

She had thought of this as a house for the defeated, the end station for bitter desperation. The other parents laughed. How could they?

Chapter Eight

It was the day before Christmas Eve. They played their way into Christmas. They were determined not to give up playing. Our little house was warm and cozy and had room for everything that was part of Christmas—ceremonial seriousness in the face of something important about to happen, expectations about packages that mustn't be opened but whose contents may be guessed at. And in the midst of it all, an open fire that breathes and pants and whose breath is mixed with the smell of sealing wax and newly cut wood.

Lisa and Patrick cut and glued small paper baskets for the Christmas tree. The stand was placed in its usual corner while awaiting the little spruce tree that would soon be bought. Daddy kept an eye on the Christmas ham that was baking while Mummy rushed around without having any clear idea of what she was actually doing.

Berit scampered about on her knees while I lay in the centre of the floor in the big room, a tiny bundle with eyes that wouldn't stay still.

Women's work give the house its character on those last days before Christmas. Children potter about. The women speak a special language of their own. Those are the best days. You work with odds and ends, wonder about things out loud and know you have a place in the scheme of things, a place you don't have to fight for. Daddy keeps out of the way.

On that afternoon he sat in front of the cooker, stared at the ham, drank beer and tried enviously to break into an intimacy that wasn't his. He refused to believe what he saw, he said. This busy idyll was contrary to Mummy's character.

He took hold of her as she rushed past the cooker and tried to pull her down onto his knee. Why didn't she have a drink with him and love him a little. Just a little.

Mummy jumped out of the way. He had to satisfy himself with staring at the ham. Although heaven only knows why he did it. It managed quite well on its own.

He gave her a smack on the bottom that made her hiss with anger.

Take care, she said.

Of what?

She made an indecent gesture. They've always been rather indecent when they joke with each other. She pointed to show him that if he didn't keep his hands off her she was going to push part of him, an important part, into the vegetable grater she had just assembled.

It's time we discussed your character, he said.

What about it?

She cranked the handle of the grater wildly.

Now you're going to listen to me, he said.

He'd never imagined her as commander-in-chief over a crowd of crazy Christmas elves, over this orgy in Christmas preparations.

You can talk, she said and abandoned the vegetable grater. She stood firmly in front of him, out of his reach and said: I think we shouldn't have any Christmas presents.

Of course we're going to have Christmas presents, he said.

She wanted to give the money to the foreign country where the barefooted soldiers in black are. Instead, he bought a stereo system.

When I met you, he said, you were a modern woman. Everyone thought you were modern and enlightened. At most, you knew how to fry frozen fish fingers.

She played his game for a while. But then the game was over as far as she was concerned. She looked past him and towards me, the spastic child, lying on the floor. She tried to recall the hopeful laughs she'd heard in the waiting room at the Centre.

Daddy noticed her disquiet. It rose like a tidal wave within her. He got up and pulled her towards him. Don't worry, he whispered.

She smiled bravely at him. What about the exercises? Were they any good? She felt she'd already forgotten the complicated movements.

We'll train Asa, we'll do exactly as we've been taught. She'll be a healthy child.

Yes, she said.

You and I.

She pressed herself against him. It comforted her. Daddy put his hand on her hip. He caressed her and wanted to play again. They should go down to the basement, just the two of them, and do nice things with each other.

He misunderstood her signals. He can be hopelessly insensitive. Her anguish hung like icicles around her heart. She tore herself free and rushed to her children. Sometimes, she says, sometimes he sounds like a dirty old man who lures little girls into the woods to drink beer.

Men! It sounded like a swear-word. There should be some way of insuring oneself against them. Or they should invent a medicine that provides lifelong protection. They're impossible beings. She thought it then and she thinks it even more now. Be careful, Asa, she says. In the morning they want a pal to read the newspaper with and discuss the doings of the world. When evening comes you're supposed to stand in front of the cooker, red-cheeked from baking, and a few hours later they expect you to transform yourself into a bomb. A sex bomb!

Men are a nuisance, she says. Most of them live in an old fantasy world in which men control everything. They don't understand that they've become superfluous. That it'll soon be time to replace them with a sperm bank.

Daddy stared listlessly at the ham through the oven

door. He didn't want to be replaced by a sperm bank. He thought that Mummy should put on something he calls her peekaboo outfit. It consists of tiny briefs, a garter belt and a bra through which her nipples poke out. Mummy should learn to bake buns and knead dough wearing her peekaboo outfit. All women should. Lisa's teacher too. Then going to parent-teacher meetings would be fun.

Men, Mummy sighed, this time in resignation. After all, she can't do without them. Lisa had already begun to look at herself in the mirror. Just the way Mummy always does, blowing her hair and putting artificial tan on her face so that she can radiate at all the men she meets.

Patrick got up, tired of making the Christmas decorations. He wanted to buy a Christmas tree.

Absolutely not, Daddy said. The time to buy a Christmas tree is on Christmas Eve. The prices go down then.

I don't want a second-hand Christmas tree, Patrick said. He leaped around the kitchen, waving his hands.

Daddy went into the livingroom and sat down beside me. I floundered helplessly with my nose against the blanket. I was completely incapable of getting my elbows under my body.

New eyes! Daddy wrote in his journal. One acquires new eyes not only because one suddenly sees the disabled children but also because one sees the healthy children in a new way.

One distinguishes a movement, a wink or a jump. One etches it on plate as though it were one of the seven wonders of the world.

Patrick danced around. I, the spastic child, couldn't turn. For a child to turn from its back to its stomach, one tiny little turn, is the result of such a complicated interaction of reflexes that all the computers in the world couldn't map out even a fraction of it. That was what Daddy wrote on the back of a picture showing me lying in the bird position. The brain is the most complicated structure known to man.

You acquire new eyes. Daddy explained how it feels.

You're split, split by a flash of lightning, split all the way through. One half of you plays the game, jokes and teases its way forward. The other half broods, goes over the same thoughts that have already been thought a hundred times, sees the child who can't . . . They had decided to start my exercises for the first time before dinner. At the Centre they had signed a receipt for the little red, wooden stick and the gym mat.

Everything an infant does is a preparation for moving, for standing up. That was what the physical therapist said. Everything collaborates, through the baby turning over from its back to its stomach, up on its elbows, up on its knees. All of it so that man will rise above the creeping lizards. Up on his feet! Up and walk!

Split by lightning, they were both condemned to be split by lightning.

§

We see, we know. Despite that we play the game. Patrick wanted something. Not a Christmas tree, something else. He wanted to buy something. Daddy sat with one hand on me, went over things with that part of his being the lightning had split off.

You're not listening, Mummy said.

What is it?

Patrick wants to buy something, she said.

Mummy thought that Patrick should be rewarded. He'd improved since he'd thrown the pizzas at the domestic science teacher and since all the meetings. Mummy had found hydraulic bolt shears hidden in the basement. That was what he used to clip off the moped locks. She threw the shears in the rubbish bin.

Patrick's marks at school were good. Before he used to get only one out of five in general subjects. Now he came home with a three.

What do you want? Daddy asked.

I want a Slush, Patrick said.
What's that? Mummy asked.
It's something bloody awful, Daddy said. Something poisonous that children drink.
It can't be very good for them, Mummy said.
Of course not, Daddy said and gave Patrick five crowns.
Well, all right, Mummy said. After all, it's Christmas. She preferred to see Patrick eat müsli. Daddy said it's the sort of thing they sweep up from the barn floors. Mummy eats it on sour milk because it makes her feel healthy.
Well, you can have a Slush, she said. You've been a good boy.
We're proud of you, Daddy said.
Pooh! Patrick said.
You've shown that you can work, Mummy said. That's the main thing. You've studied.
Studied what? Patrick seemed genuinely surprised.
Your homework of course, Daddy said. You've improved your marks to a three.
Pooh! Patrick said again.
But you must have done something, Mummy said. She thought Patrick seemed embarassed. There's no need to be modest. What did you do to improve your marks?
Nothing, Patrick said. I haven't said anything and I haven't done anything for an entire term. That's why I got a three.
He bounded out through the door on his way towards the sweet shop where the owner, an old blood-sucker, had built himself a nest from which he bombarded the area with Sour Bombs and Slush.

§

My parents are comedians. They themselves don't understand the full extent of their comedy. I think of an old film and of them as two Laurel and Hardy types, constantly subjected to shocks of surprise.

It's like sitting watching a slapstick film in a trench. I've seen a Chaplin film on video. Chaplin is in the war. The film runs a little too quickly, they all move with jerky movements.

The screams are real. The screams from those hanging on the barbed wire out there, from me, Asa.

Aunt Tilly was almost knocked down by Patrick rushing out to buy his Slush. She carried her bags in over the threshold. One by one the circles of intimacy were broken. Lisa sat alone with the Christmas decorations. She gave up and played for a while with Berit. The enchantment disintegrated.

Mummy looked unhappy. Daddy helped Aunt Tilly off with her rustling raincoat.

How's Asa? Aunt Tilly asked.

She left her bags in the hall. She'd dredged through the city flea markets. Lisa fished up three German beer cans with Father Christmas on them.

Daddy's stomach protested. Soon he'd have to go to the lavatory. His stomach was dissolving.

Welcome, Aunt Tilly said and went into the big room.

We're going to put Asa through exercises, Daddy said.

What's wrong with her?

She's disabled, Daddy said.

In what way?

Daddy didn't answer. That was going to become a habit with him. People walk up to you on the street and say hello and ask how you are. Everything's fine, you say, we're really fine except one of the kids happens to be spastic. No, you just can't say it, not like that.

So she's spastic, Aunt Tilly said.

Lisa came into the room with Berit creeping after her. Lisa showed a porcelain dog she'd found amongst Aunt Tilly's treasures.

Look, she said and held out the dog.

You can have it in your room, Mummy said quickly. I

thought it could stand there, Aunt Tilly said. In the window.

Daddy felt as though his stomach was going to explode. He tried to hold off the attack. He wanted to go up to the lavatory and sit there with his car ads. But he had to stay. He was the commander on a drifting ship. He had to stay to ward off a major accident.

Aunt Tilly sank down on the sofa. I was still lying on the floor. Berit crept up to me and began to play with my toes. Aunt Tilly's thin bones creaked when she sat down. Daddy heard her. For the first time he heard her body ageing. I, the spastic child on the floor, made her older.

I see, Aunt Tilly said. How sad.

Here it comes, Daddy thought. He knew her, he'd grown up with her laments. When he came home with poor marks from school or when he broke his leg, it was a pity about him, but it was more of a pity about Aunt Tilly. And wasn't it really a pity about her now, having this happen to her. Asa!

Daddy thought he knew her but he was wrong. She sat in silence for a while with her groaning joints. Then she bent forward and pulled me up from the floor. She hugged me. She sat a while and rocked me slowly. The only thing wrong was her eyes, the desperate expression in them! Oh, I know. I know what they said and how they looked at me. Asa'll never get better!

She can be trained out of her disablement, Daddy said.

He began to explain. But he was far too nervous for it to make any sense. While the nerves are still growing in a child's brain, new wiring can be run past the wires that are burnt out. He wasn't sure Aunt Tilly was listening.

But she was listening all right. Aunt Tilly hears and sees everything, even when she's grieving. She registered their anguish, she went over their territory with a minesweeper.

What wiring are you talking about? she said and looked at Daddy as though the accident had deprived him of his wits.

Is that what they said at the Centre? That you should change the wiring in Asa's brain?

Not exactly. But that's how I understood it.

Aunt Tilly thought they should all have a cup of coffee. She didn't want to hear about wiring anymore.

I have to clean up, Mummy said.

We're expecting visitors, Daddy said.

Mummy tore down the Chinese posters from the walls and dried the floor. She'd put an ad in the papers for help. There was no question of a day nursery, not now that I was to be put through the exercises four times a day.

Are you going to work? Aunt Tilly asked and rocked me on her knee.

Yes, Mummy said.

No, Aunt Tilly said.

She has to, Daddy said. We need the money.

He left them. His stomach had become a divebomber. The bomb flaps were about to open. At the bottom of the stairs he began to unbutton his trousers.

Surely you can see that you must stay at home, Aunt Tilly said.

Why? Mummy said.

Can't you see that?

Mummy took me from Aunt Tilly and put me in an armchair. She picked up Berit. Her children gave her a feeling of independence.

We'll be able to handle this, Mummy said. If we can just get help.

I can move here, Aunt Tilly said.

No thank you, Mummy said. We've put an ad in the papers.

Is it for the money? Is it really for the money?

We'll talk about that later, Mummy said.

I can help you. Aunt Tilly opened her bag. She dug out a bankbook. I can lend you money.

The WC on the floor above flushed. The pipe from the

WC runs down behind the thin wall of the living room. You can hear the water flush down.

It's very kind of you, Mummy said. But we don't need to borrow money.

She left the room. She took her children away from Aunt Tilly. Absolutely not, she thought. Half the things in the livingroom had been supplied by Aunt Tilly. Aunt Tilly had thrown iron chains around them. They already had a debt. It pulled them down. You have to be an escape artist to get out.

Mummy didn't understand Aunt Tilly. That's what Daddy says. They didn't have a single thought in common. Aunt Tilly came from a world where people have to stick together. Daddy explained and Mummy became irritated. Did he mean she didn't want them to stick together?

Not in that way. No one handed out help in the area where Aunt Tilly was born. There you had to stick together. That was the only important thing. Those who didn't stick together perished. If you haven't experienced it you can never understand it.

Mummy came from another world. You don't have to be rich in that world, not by any means. But the safety net is always there. People who know people, names that sound familiar, the invisible language that no one has succeeded in describing.

Aunt Tilly sat abandoned on the sofa. With her thin fingers she opened up her bank-book. The bank-book contained the meagre savings of her lifetime. Take what I have. She would have been capable of cutting off her right hand if necessary. If only she could be of use, if only she could buy herself a place amongst the living, buy herself free from her solitude in the stone desert of the city.

At that moment there was a knock on the door. The bell was broken, it had been broken when they moved into the house. Daddy had drawn up a plan for how it should be repaired. A yearly plan.

The short hours of daylight had gone. Out there on the

steps stood Elsa, old Elsa. My story leads her to our door. Elsa and Aunt Tilly! My story brings them together, the city and the darkness let go of them and place them on the steps in front of our house, the way abandoned children were placed on the church steps in the old days.

Mummy opened the door and was surprised by Elsa's appearance. Elsa was wearing a uniform, a dark-blue cape, a white starched collar, white cuffs, an apron and the emblem, the proud emblem of her profession, needled in position under her chin. He clothes were newly ironed. She looked perfect.

It's about the ad, she said.

Come in! Mummy said.

She'd expected someone different, someone ordinary, any sort of a someone except this sort. People don't go around in uniform nowadays. It's ages since anybody did it in child welfare. The house, like everybody in it, drew a deep breath.

Aunt Tilly looked out from the dreadful sofa. What she saw made her happy. Elsa's uniform was a guarantee of expertise. And expertise costs money. Now, at any rate, they were going to need help. She put the bank-book back down into her handbag without feeling envious.

Mummy went up the stairs first. Inside her she struggled against her disappointment. They'd never be able to afford it. A proper children's nurse must have proper wages. What had she expected? Everybody needs proper wages.

She showed Elsa the room. It looks a little untidy, she said, talking the way women usually do. In fact she'd cleaned the room and, as usual when she cleans up, she'd filled the house with martyred cries. Daddy'd helped her. They'd cleaned off the dirt from the mouldings, even from the edges that couldn't be seen.

As I say, it's a little untidy, Mummy said, but that's because of the Christmas rush.

It'll be all right, Elsa said.

She spoke with an accent. At first Daddy thought she

was from what he calls the whiners' belt between Norrköping and Örebro. But he was wrong. Elsa came from SmÅland, she had her whitening hair tied in a knot behind her head and she was a member of the Pentacostal Movement. She was small and round, she blinked with her short-sighted light-blue eyes at our beds and at the full-length curtains Mummy had sewn.

After no more than a few minutes Mummy felt it, there was no need to be afraid of Elsa. Despite her uniform. They were already talking as though Elsa were a member of the family.

We have a disabled child, Daddy said. Asa is disabled.

I'll help you, Elsa said.

They sat at the kitchen table. Elsa was a nice person, maybe she was even a good person. Mummy regretted having shown her the house. She regretted having spent time at it. Because now they had to talk about money and when they did it would all prove impossible.

Patrick came in. He went up to Elsa, shook hands with her and bowed formally. Lisa helped to serve the coffee and cake. It was as though the children had become participants in a great and serious ceremony.

And your wages? Mummy asked. What wages are you asking?

Elsa took out a big, white envelope. She had her life in that envelope, the proof of her skills.

This is my certificate, she said, the certificate from my training. And here are the recommendations.

They looked politely through her papers. They couldn't very well push them aside. But her wages?

I've served in hospitals, Elsa said. And I've worked for distinguished people.

You probably know everything about children, Daddy said.

Yes, Elsa said and you could see how proud she became. You could see it in the way she sat, her seriousness. I know almost everything.

And your wages?

That's not important, Elsa said.

Now you could hear the candles burning and the snow that had begun to fall outside the windows. Everything was absolutely silent in the kitchen. Aunt Tilly closed her eyes. She was suspicious. There must be something wrong with this. Wages were always important.

I've got an early retirement pension, Elsa said.

We must pay you something, Daddy said. We have to know how much.

I have a dog. A little poodle. He's called Putte. Can I have him here?

Yes, Elsa, you can have him here.

My legs aren't good and I don't see so well. You'll have to drive me sometimes.

We'll drive you. Tell us how much you want to be paid, tell us now, Elsa.

My parents are magnetic. They attract those the city rejects, those who wait without hope. It wasn't just the man with the bag or the chap who thought he was a cock. It wasn't just Aunt Tilly. Now it was old Elsa who'd come home to them to swap her services for a little consolation.

I don't know for sure what it was she saw in them, in us. It was something, something that almost made her cry at the thought that they might not be able to afford her.

She needed them. Accept me! At last they got her to mention the modest sum she wanted. They tried to increase it but it was impossible.

What are you doing for Christmas, Elsa? Mummy asked.

I'm staying at home, Elsa said. Putte and I are staying at home. We'll watch TV.

You're going to spend Christmas alone?

Yes, I'm alone.

Would you like to spend it with us?

Aunt Tilly emptied the bags that were still standing out in the hall. Jealousy gnawed at her guts. They didn't need her bank-book. They didn't need her.

At last the snow fell. It was a couple of days before Christmas. It was a day that belongs to women. It was the day when my exercises were to start, the very first exercises.

§

There's something wrong with my story here. Actually it was on Christmas Eve they first put me through my exercises. Maybe they delayed it at the last moment.

From their diaries I can see that it was Christmas Eve because Granny was there. More snow fell during the night, when the houses awoke the district was white and playing children tumbled like bear cubs in the snow. The snow ploughs didn't come that day. The cars made tracks ten centimetres deep in the snow.

Daddy went with Lisa and Patrick to fetch the Christmas tree. It was the last tree left. It was crooked and they got it for nothing. Daddy said Christmas trees don't have to be straight. He thought it was beautiful.

The bells from the little church sounded different through the snow. The candles burnt, the shepherds sang the praises of the Child, Patrick got a hockey set and Lisa got a doll's house.

They placed the red-green gym mat on the table in the living room, right up beside the tiled stove. That's where it would lie for a year. It became a battleground in their war against nature, against the mistakes nature had made.

They took off my clothes. Aunt Tilly, Granny and Elsa sat beside the window. Elsa had Putte in her lap. Stay where you are, Daddy said. You're not disturbing us.

He wanted to show them. It wasn't dangerous, it was an adventure. They placed me on the mat. Daddy put the little wooden stick in my hand and carefully pressed forward my head. I began to scream. Mummy stood beside him. She tried to help by holding me. My scream made her uncertain. Daddy too became uncertain. How was it they were supposed to hold me?

The physical therapist had shown them. It had seemed so simple and clear. They were to hold me in the creeping position. But how should my legs be?

I screamed more loudly.

One of the women dropped a coffee cup. Coffee ran out over the white tablecloth. Coffee dripped down onto the floor.

Daddy worked with me. His big hands were gentle. Don't hurt her, don't use any force at all! But his hands were also clumsy. I screamed. Do we have to do it on Christmas Eve? Mummy said.

When are we going to do it otherwise?

Tomorrow.

That's Christmas Day.

Mummy had to raise her voice to make herself heard above my screams. She thought they should wait. No, there was no waiting. The first step had been taken. The contract had been signed. They were moving out amongst the extinguished stars. They'd become aware of life, the life that slowly stiffens and dies. The life that can be awakened, the paths that can be put to use.

If we turn back now, it's the end. There's only one chance. There's only one time and that time is now! If we let the days pass they'll carry her with them. They'll twist her, they'll nail her to her illness.

We can't begin the exercises with an excuse for not doing them, Daddy said.

The old women got up. Elsa muttered something about not wanting to disturb. They left the room. Aunt Tilly's sad eyes gleamed in the doorway. Those are the eyes I still have fixed on me. Asa'll never get better.

Granny, too, left me, abandoned me. She was the one who could have helped.

Why don't you stop them?

Because they're your parents.

Don't you hear me?

They're doing what they think is right.

My screams should move you to tears. How can you remain untouched!

I'm not untouched.

Why are you going then?

They closed the door behind them. They sat in the kitchen and listened to my screams.

Help me, Daddy said. We can start it gently, Mummy said.

I'm being gentle, Daddy said. I'm touching her as though she were a butterfly. Help me.

We don't need to put her through any more exercises now, Mummy said. She must get used to it.

He was on his knees at the table. He held me. Asa isn't going to get used to it. What we're touching is what's sick inside her. She's screaming to retain the sickness. You have to help me. We must do this together.

They tried again. They put together the grips they had learned. Daddy tried to ring the physical therapist at home. It was Christmas Eve. He heard the telephone line crackle desolately. At the other end was nothing.

They put me through the exercises with the single thought of not giving up. You direct your gaze towards a tiny point far away. You walk towards that point and you refuse to let yourself look to either side. If you look to either side for too long you lose your balance.

The old women sat in the kitchen. The radio played Christmas songs. Patrick was out in the snow with his hockey set. Lisa was furnishing her doll's house. Granny left them. She needed fresh air, she said. She went on a Christmas Eve walk.

Aunt Tilly and old Elsa could find nothing to distract their minds. A struggle they didn't understand was in full sway in the room beside them. Aunt Tilly picked at things on the table. Her hands couldn't rest.

I know what they thought and what they felt. It gradually emerged from them. I know what evil spirits glared at them from the corners of the room.

There's no help for the crippled. And there's no point imagining there is either.

Aunt Tilly defended herself against what she saw. Inside her she saw the Home. As a child she'd lived for a while on the north side of the city. There, just outside the old city limits, was the Home, a place of terror, the very deepest layer of fear. The Home was surrounded by a tall fence. You couldn't look in. You shouldn't look in.

The fence protected the city. Images of those who were inside flourished. Notions of the abnormal, the crippled who were brought there because no one could stand to look at them. It was so awful that anyone who saw had a thorn in his eye for the rest of his life.

There were boys who dared look. They climbed up on the fence. They looked in. They said they saw grunting beings with twisted legs. The idiots, they shouted. We can see the idiots!

The bravest amongst them threw sticks and stones. The children squealed with the delight wakened by terror and by the forbidden. When the gates were opened and they were sent packing, they withdrew imitating what they'd seen, grunting, beside themselves with giggles.

Things got better, Elsa said.

Aunt Tilly nodded but without any conviction. They made detours around the Home. They still did it during the 1940s. The taxi drivers refused to drive in through the gates. What could be seen in there was too awful. The doctors had to get out of the taxis outside the gates and walk in.

Elsa looked out through the kitchen window. She'd have preferred to think of something else. A thousand pinpricks of light gleamed in the snow. In all the gardens people had hung out little lamps. The treetops sparkled with light. Her heart beat faster. She heard a hymn, her hymn being sung on the radio. She turned up the volume. A star shines wonderously clear.

How she remembered! She remembered more than Aunt Tilly, who only had the blurred terrors of the streets for company. When Elsa was training as a nurse she visited the Home. They walked in a group through the huge dormitories. They kept close together to give each other strength. It was like a barracks. The children sat beside porcelain sinks and washed themselves.

She saw children who lay tied to their beds. Their legs were brittle, she was told. They had to be tied down so that they didn't fall out of bed. She remembered the sleepless nights she spent after she had visited the Home.

But things got better. She remembered the two children, the poster with the two children who reached up towards heaven. There was going to be a search for the hidden children. One child was red, the other, the forgotten child, was black.

They began to search. There was a big campaign. The women sat with their memories. Aunt Tilly's restless hands wandered down into her handbag. She took our a handkerchief and blew her nose. She didn't look at Elsa. Her eyes were fixed on the dark corners of her memory. Her eyes were bitter at the savage fate that had struck down another human being.

That was in the 1950s. They found crippled children in old people's homes. They found them in calf pens and in cellars. They were kept out of sight when visitors came. The shame of it! Aunt Tilly put her handkerchief back into her handbag. The shame of having a child like that! How is one to become free of the family's shame of its disabled member, of what is born with neither purpose nor meaning?

I don't think Aunt Tilly herself felt any shame. It would be unfair to say that. She was sad, so pitch-black in her sadness and in her conviction that what had been born crippled must remain crippled.

It was only fifteen years ago, Elsa said. They'd already sent up a Sputnik when the last children were brought up from the cellars.

The two women sat in the caressing fragrances of Christmas Eve, frightened by their memories and my cries, Asa's lamentations. The little poodle whimpered in Elsa's lap and Lisa talked to herself and her doll's house.

They found the hidden children. They gave them light and love. I'd stopped screaming. Can one do more? Can one rectify what's happened? They didn't think so.

Granny came in with snow on her shoes. She'd walked past the church. She'd stood outside and heard the singing. A child is born! She'd looked in through the colourful windows and sensed the shadow of Christ on the cross.

Granny opened the door to the living room. I hung sobbing in Mummy's arms. It was Christmas Eve and time for children to celebrate.

Chapter Nine

Soon it will be morning. I whisper it in the solitude of my room. I kiss my rabbit's nose and feel the touch of what is alive. The feeling remains on my lips, even when I move away.

I can sense what it feels like to touch one's child.

My story runs ahead of me, and points out what happened. I don't say they were wrong. When I curse their presumption it's my resisting body that curses. I interpret my cries. Then I was a seven-kilo Asa with a consciousness that was just beginning. I don't say the doctor from Prague was wrong. Who am I to judge the medical aspects of it?

I must enter into my story. I can't explain it any better than that. When morning comes you'll know what happened to me. And to them. It's up to you. Judge, if you want to.

I kiss my rabbit and know how they touched me. Not the way parents normally touch their children. They took off all their clothes except their underpants. They held me. They stood naked with their spastic child. They climbed up on the table with the gym mat.

They were so careful. They wanted to be sure there wasn't a single edge that could chafe, not a single button that could tear.

They acted like giants, fairytale giants who find the most fragile of things and hold it in their giant hands. They took hold of what was to be held in me. They rolled over me. They were as soft as the softest cloth. They never squeezed or forced. They were walruses that play and snort in the sea.

My mouth against the rabbit's nose, their skin against mine. Their bodies fused together with my body. Our suffering became a suffering in common.

I wish my story had a soul. I wish its soul was in the feeling that's left when you've touched what is alive.

If only morning would come. If only I could sleep. My story is approaching the point where my cries were mixed with their's. I see defeat approach.

I've never been awake an entire night. I've never been so tired. The pages with the case records shine in front of me on the desk. If only I dared I'd burn them up in the stove. Now it was winter and the city shook it's dishevelled hair. Snow and January winds in the treetops. The snow embankments grew bigger along the street outside our house. Daddy bought a heater to keep the car engine warm and another heater to put inside the car so that it wouldn't be cold when they drove me into town.

Once a week they drove to the Centre. They began to feel at home in the waiting room. They stopped being surprised that spastic kids can laugh and be rowdy. Again they met the woman and the child they had met on their first visit.

She lived in Paris. Every month she came with her boy to the Centre in Stockholm.

Will he get better? Mummy asked.

The woman smiled. Her boy had been completely slack. Like a rag. Now he could sit up in his pram. There'd been something, a fibre, a path that could be used.

A waiting room for the hopeful! They almost forgot their desperation. The physical therapist helped them, corrected the errors they'd made. They manipulated my body with more confidence.

But they saw no improvement.

It takes more than a few weeks, the physical therapist said.

Why does Asa scream like that?

The physical therapist had no answer. I screamed more than other children. They'd just have to try to put up with it. In her abrupt way she informed them of new observations. My disability was becoming more and more apparent. Now it could be seen quite clearly.

Their confidence in the physical therapist grew. Her unshakable authority gave them the calm they needed.

Life was arranged to suit the exercises and our trips to the Centre. Mummy and Daddy shared the days between them. The exercises took time. And they didn't just want to do the exercises. They wanted to play with me and talk to me. After the exercises they had to comfort me.

I screamed but I wasn't getting any better.

They had Elsa. She worked hard and she was efficient. She knew tricks for everything. She made carrot purées for stomachs that were out of order, she knew of ointments and ways for curing red bottoms and colds in the head. When Mummy and Daddy opened the door to our room we lay there like two rose-hip flowers, newly bathed, packed down, in clean, freshly ironed sheets.

Elsa filled the house and the kitchen with her art. With magic hands she conjured up meatballs and crisp sprat-and-potato pies. She didn't have to do it. At first they were embarrassed. But it was her gift to them. She wanted to show them, to make them happy.

Elsa's poodle, Putte, lay growling under the kitchen table. Putte was nervous and shivery. Mummy's never liked dogs. She liked Putte about as much as she would have liked a psychopath with a razor. Poodles are the worst, she says.

Putte bit her in the leg.

Ah! she screamed.

Shame, Putte! Elsa said.

Why does he bite? Mummy said.

He's guarding my handbag, Elsa said.

Putte had made red marks in Mummy's plump white legs. Elsa fetched cottonwool and disinfectant.

You might get blood poisoning, she said in a worried voice.

Daddy wondered which of them would get the blood poisoning, Putte or Mummy.

You should go to hospital, he said, as he grinned. The casualty department. Being bitten by a dog is a serious matter. You must have an anti-tetanus injection.

Mummy looked angry.

Daddy began to teach her dog psychology. A dog senses immediately if you're inferior. That's when it bites. You must take command of a dog.

He bent down under the table. Putte sat there growling. Daddy stretched out his hand. Putte bit him.

Ouch! Daddy cried. Damn it!

Shame, Putte, Elsa said again.

It was worst for Berit. She crept along the floor like a tiny streak of lightning. Putte marked out his territory and when Berit entered it he nipped her. This battle went on all the time Putte was with us.

Elsa grew unhappy. One morning she rang and said she couldn't come. She slurred her words. At last it emerged, her secret affliction.

She took pills. Sometimes she drank.

I think she's hooked on pills, Mummy said.

She takes medicine because she's in pain, Daddy said.

She's in pain because of the medicine, Mummy said. She's becoming blind.

Elsa stayed at home when she was tipsy. Mummy drove over to her flat and talked with her. Elsa had been in hospital. They ran electric currents through her. It's called electro-shock treatment.

Sometimes she took the ferry boat to Finland, to Åland. She had three women friends and she went off with them. They smuggled. They hid bottles in their corsets and in all the folds of their bodies.

There were a lot of folds, Daddy says.

When Elsa had been to Åland with her gang of smugglers she was always absent a few days.

Those Åland trips aren't good for you, Mummy said.

There aren't many pleasures in life, Elsa said.

What does your church say? Mummy said. After all, you're a member of the Pentacostal Movement.

I don't take the Pentacostal Movement with me to Åland, Elsa said.

They needed her. I don't think Elsa was ever tipsy when she was with us. Mummy was overjoyed at being able to work again. She went to her Celestial Wardrobe to design new clothes.

But my screams began to wear them down. Mummy had regained her liberty, but she wasn't free. The weeks passed and they could see no improvement.

My screams pursued them. I was screaming more loudly now. They began to worry about the neighbours. My screams could be heard out in the street.

The physical therapist explained that a lot of people don't succeed with the exercises. They can't keep it up. They begin to cheat. The husband ends up putting the child through them on his own. His wife leaves the room, puts on the vacuum cleaner to avoid hearing.

We mustn't cheat, Daddy said.

He became irritated with Elsa. She cluttered about or started the mixer in the kitchen when it was time for my exercises.

He took up the matter with her. You know that we must put Asa through those exercises.

I know that, she said.

You don't have to raise hell in the kitchen every time.

I shan't do it anymore, she said with the sort of voice she must once have used when she served rich masters.

The next time Daddy put me through the exercises she made more noise than ever.

As long as we don't cheat, Daddy said to Mummy. Promise me that.

Mummy promised. They were going to share it.

But the exercises wore them down. It affected their moods. The worst was that there was no change, that my state remained stationary.

Lisa became jealous again. She dreamt of putting me in the rubbish bin.

§

I try to imagine how they marched into their defeat without knowing it. Afterwards you can see it. Afterwards you've learned.

But it's at this time you need to grasp it.

Life is like that, Daddy says. You can't get away from it.

One feels so unsure about it all, Mummy says. She says that when Patrick was small she read fairytales to him each evening. He liked fairytales. Afterwards she lay silent and motionless beside him to help him fall asleep.

But Patrick didn't want to fall asleep. Mummy was twenty-four then and was worried about Patrick. She wanted him to feel secure.

She lay beside him for hours. When she thought he was asleep she carefully lifted one leg over the edge of the bed. Patrick would sit up at once. Wide awake. What are you doing, Mummy? he asked.

Then she'd lay there for another hour. But every time she started to get up he was awake.

For two years she lay beside him at least four hours every night. Life became a nightmare, she says.

Mummy and Patrick's father divorced, Daddy says. No one can stand a child like that and a mother like that.

Why did you do it? Patrick asks. He likes to hear her talk about it. Although it embarasses him as well.

I think I felt guilty, Mummy says.

Guilty about what?

I don't know. Perhaps many mothers feel a sort of guilt for their children. About not being adequate. About bringing them into a life that will harm them.

What happened? Patrick asks.

I went to a psychologist, Mummy says.

Ugh, Daddy says.

A good psychologist, Mummy says.

The psychologist advised her to put Patrick to bed at half past eight, to kiss him goodnight, to say now it's time to sleep, and then to leave the room.

And you did it? Patrick says.

Yes, Mummy nods. The first time I almost collapsed with nervousness.

And what happened?

You fell asleep at once, of course, Mummy says.

She's calculated that, in the preceding years, she lay over three thousand hours beside Patrick. Unnecessarily. She learnt. Could she make use of that knowledge now when she put me through my exercises, me the spastic child?

They mapped out the days and weeks. Things weren't going to be like they were with Patrick. Every minute became as precious as gold. Everything that had to be done was given its own little compartment.

They invited friends around. They wanted to show how competent and clever they were. They wanted to be praised. But there were people who almost choked over how competent and clever they were.

Mostly new mothers, Daddy says. New mothers who make the old mistakes. Who complain about one child taking too much time.

It's not as simple as that, Mummy says.

New mothers can be lethal, Daddy says. Particularly if they have compliant husbands. They go dotty with all the attention they give their child and they get dotty children.

You talk too much, Mummy says.

Her political friends came to our place and read from their little red books. On Saturdays they stood with boxes and collected money for foreign countries. They stood in the snow outside the old Co-operative shop and rattled their boxes.

Mummy discovered that there was a shortage of day nurseries in the district. She immediately organized a group of mothers. They got in touch with the local politicians.

You were terrific, Daddy says. Although he doesn't sound happy when he says it. As though the events had given his memories a bitter flavour.

Mummy stopped being chairman of the PTA. It was because of the business about Lisa.

You do what you think is right, she says.

One day Lisa saw a few boys hit a smaller boy in the playground. Two teachers were strolling past. But they looked the other way. They didn't want to bother. Lisa went up to the teachers. She gave them a piece of her mind.

Of course I did, Lisa says. She still gets angry when she thinks about it. You should see her when she's angry. Her eyes flash. I don't know anyone who looks fiercer than she does.

They thought you were cheeky, Mummy says.

Of course I was cheeky, Lisa says. Lazy teachers get cheeky pupils.

She was a little tot when it happened and little tots have no right to speak. She was reported. Then she was forced to apologize to the teachers for behaving badly.

Wasn't I right? Lisa says.

Why did you apologize then? Patrick says.

Lisa turns her head away. The light in her eyes goes out. Mummy takes her hand and strokes it. Sometimes it doesn't help being right.

You learn. Mummy and Daddy thought they'd mastered the difficult art of living. They thought they'd learnt and that they knew how. They had their beloved house and Elsa who took care of everyday life. They had each other and their unshakable trust. Things couldn't have been better.

If it weren't for me. And for the fact that I wasn't improving.

§

It can begin invisibly. You don't notice. Not at first. You're steady as a house with heavy feet. No need to bother about small currents of water that push at the foundations and tickle you around your toes.

That was how their doubts began.

The physical therapist received them with her patience and her abrupt explanations. Of course the exercises were showing results.

I became restless as soon as we got to the steps leading to the Centre. As soon as I saw the physical therapist I began to cry. I grew frightened of white coats. Many years afterwards white coats still made me uneasy. I remember the first time we were to go to the National Dental Clinic. There was so many things wrong with me, not only my eyes and my thumbs but also my teeth. They grew crookedly.

When I saw the dentist's white coat I gave a cry, the sort of cry that cracks glass. Daddy promised me a telescope. He thought a telescope would calm me. Berit was green with envy.

How you go on with Asa! Berit still says it when she feels neglected. Asa got a telescope just to go to the dentist.

The physical therapist used my body to show them. It was more difficult to talk now since I made so much noise.

The exercises are beginning to stabilize her, the physical therapist said.

Asa's working, just look how she's working. It's not just her free leg that kicks when she's held down. Asa's working with her pelvis and her shoulders. We're holding her but we're not locking her. We're giving her a sturdy position from which to fight.

They nodded obediently. I fought like one possessed.

They tried to see what the physical therapist said she saw. But they didn't notice any improvement.

The dogged monotony, the constant repetition of a rigid schedule that couldn't be changed . . . It takes enormous strength. Doubts undermined them. Decisions that had once been solid as cast concrete now showed cracks, bits crumbled away, the ground began to soften.

They'd never have admitted it. Not then. Doubt was not a guest at their table. Elsa clattered. I screamed.

Daddy began to devote more time to me. He came home earlier. He stayed at home for longer and longer after the exercises.

He should have given more time to his theater. He worked at his new play. He used the tricks he'd learned. Old tricks. He should have thought out new ones. His hands wrote while he was absent.

His spirit was with me. Everything was concentrated on my exercises and on the fact that something must soon happen. People began to wonder about him.

What wore him down couldn't be seen. His hands became more efficient than ever. His typewriter was white hot when he wrote. He was a man who did his duty. He became a dutiful writer.

For no reason he told people to go to hell. He couldn't sit still when he talked to people. He was distracted in everything he did except this dogged writing. And my exercises!

He had friends who warned him. Things were getting out of hand.

He shrugged. It would work out.

Nothing works out by itself. People advised him to give more time to the Rabble. After all, he liked them. But he grew more and more fed up with them.

They'll change, he said. The actor who gets the leading part will change first. That's what they're like, easily led. They'll change when they see the box office figures. How many people came to see the last play? Thirty thousand!

Listen to us, his friends told him. Think of what you're saying. Otherwise.

Not even then did he bother about them. He mouthed a few curses. His mind was elsewhere.

It was with me. It wasn't a matter of choice. He was pushed in front of me and the gym mat by forces he wasn't yet aware of. Now, afterwards, it becomes obvious. You can see it in the pictures in the album I have on my desk. How doubt begins to wear out the carefree look in his eyes.

The ground dissolved around their feet. Those who begin to doubt must hold on. Their grip tightens.

He reached a deadlock. Mummy's hinted at it. His ambitions and his will were as tense as the muscles in my body.

Mummy noticed it. She moved over to him at night as he lay there with his eyes open, staring at the ceiling. Those who have slept for a long time side by side know when the other is awake. She heard and she wanted to dissolve the knot inside him.

What is it?

You know what it is, he said.

What are you talking about?

She didn't want to talk. She let her hand slide amongst the bedclothes and over his body. That was what she wanted.

He moved away.

We can't think about Asa all the time, she said.

No, he said and sat on one corner of the bed. He seemed frozen. He would have moved even further off from her if the wall hadn't been in the way.

You're too ambitious, she said.

He didn't answer. He just sat there, with a head that had become too big and that grew heavier and heavier with all his thoughts of me, the spastic child.

Come here, she whispered.

What do you mean we can't think of Asa all the time? He spoke with a voice that jangled. You mean we should cut down the exercises?

I didn't say that.

What are you trying to say then?

She sighed and rolled back, away from him. He felt her hand leave his body and felt how his body grew cold where her hand had rested. They lay there like that listening to each other's wakefulness. He had searched for betrayal in her. The beginning of betrayal. He no longer trusted her.

It was something new, a new fear that followed her into sleep.

He lay awake that night and several other nights. I can imagine Aunt Tilly's eyes and how she regards him as he lies there.

Now, too, as I sit here in my room I can see those eyes. Morning is on its way. I put Aunt Tilly on the windowsill out there. My story reminds me of what her eyes have to say. That child will never be healthy!

Daddy can't have avoided noticing her lack of faith. But she never said a word of criticism. If she had said anything he would have closed the door for ever.

He made new, unsuccessful attempts to show her. Look at what we're doing! Try to understand!

Aunt Tilly nodded but her eyes were empty because of what she couldn't understand.

Asa's improving, she muttered obediently.

Look for yourself, Daddy said.

They both looked. Mummy's face hovered in the background like an indistinct, uneasy patch.

The physical therapist says she's getting better. He laughed confidently but it was a confidence he didn't feel.

He should have paid more attention to other things. He was locked in doubt. You could make a catalogue of all the things he should have devoted himself to. He should have gone skating with Lisa. He should have gone skiing.

The snow was almost a metre deep around the city. It was a season of sunny Sundays. People set off on skis with oranges and thermoses. Children swirled down the slopes on round sledges.

Mummy tried to get him to go out. He didn't want to. He was too restless. Please, she said. For my sake.

No, not even for her sake. He neglected them.

Mummy spent a whole day preparing the skis, the ski poles, the boots for Lisa and Patrick. She'd got in touch with a girlfriend. They were going to go skiing together with the children. The preparations turned out to be troublesome, as you'll know if you've ever tried to adjust old-fashioned bindings without any tools. It was Daddy's fault. He's always talking about the need for a man in the house. But it's just talk. He didn't get any tools and he didn't help them. Mummy tried to unscrew the bindings with her fingernails and finally decided to nail Lisa's ski boots to the skis.

That's a lie, Mummy says. That story's turned into a myth. Of course I didn't nail her boots to the skis.

You tied them down with string, Patrick says.

Mummy wanted to do cross-country skiing. She says it's good for you. Patrick told me what it was like. It was dreadful, he says. They dress you up in thermally insulated one-piece suits and after a hundred metres you're drenched in sweat. The skis slip backwards. They always slip backwards. People should ski backwards.

Lisa fell all the time and got snow inside her clothes. The two women were red in the face from the effort. Everyone had frozen feet. Lisa cried. Her skis fell off. Mummy had used paper twine that broke. Lisa lay in a snow drift two kilometres inside the forest. She refused to move. A taxi, she cried. Ring for a taxi.

Lisa is a child of the city. When she was small she wanted to hear a fairy tale about a hare that hated the countryside and lived behind a rubbish bin in a backyard.

They quarrelled all the way home. Daddy got out of the way when they arrived. That was his mistake. He should have been with them that day.

But it was because of me. Me, all the time, and the questions that never led to any understandable answers. He'd ask the physical therapist if they shouldn't do more exercises with me. She was against it. Four half hours a day was already a lot. It wasn't the quantity that was important. What was important was what happened in my brain. Sometimes ten minutes could be enough.

But why wasn't I getting better?

Chapter Ten

They should have protected their idyll. They should have built walls around it and hidden themselves in each other. Here in our house they had their moments of love and the strength that consolation gives.

Outside the walls waited a world that would take the first opportunity to grind their hopes under its heel. Make mush of them. But how were they to know? Flutes played in Mummy's heart when she was able to get out and work. Despite her worry. Sitting at home too much stifles you. She needed new impressions. Particularly now that Daddy seemed so locked inside himself. He magnified things that needed to be reduced.

Work gave her moments of forgetfulness, the work in the shop, the professional questions that needed an immediate answer, the city with its bustling life and its people who didn't care in the least about a kid called Asa.

They'd been doing exercises with me for a month. It must have been at the end of January when she walked through the slushy street snow with white smoke blowing out of her mouth and her coat pulled tightly about her. She felt the winter bite around her nose and saw the tug-boats butt against the ice floes all the way into the innermost bays of the city.

There are moments when you feel so happy you sing as you walk along the street. Perhaps it was precisely that happiness that made a victim of her.

She sat in a soft armchair at Daddy's theater and waited for him. She chatted with one of the employees in the theater, a man who wrote music for the plays. She'd brought her happiness with her, the frosty splendour of the city, she'd carried it in through the door. She wasn't prepared.

How's Asa doing? the composer asked.

We put her through exercises, Mummy said.

I know, he said.

He looked worried. He'd been in our place and heard me scream.

Is it really the right thing to do? he said.

We think so, she said.

It must be painful for her, he said. I'd never be able to torment my child like that.

She was so deep inside her former self, inside the walk that had made her almost dizzy with happiness, that she didn't altogether hear what he said. He sounded so considerate. How can parents torment their child like that?

Mummy tried to describe the feeling she had. She says it's like when an entire lake suddenly freezes in front of your eyes. It creaks and at once it's frozen all the way down. Or like when you get burnt. Third degree burns. Her skin was burnt off and she was being led forward to something that consisted of more fire.

Asa's getting physical therapy, she said. The method's been tested.

Is she getting any better?

We hope so.

Most of it came out as a mumble. She should have bent forward and given him a kiss. Be careful with me. We can become so fragile. You're not really a wicked person.

I'd never do it, he repeated. I'd rather let my child stay handicapped. I'd rather that than torment her.

Mummy grabbed hold of her things and ran. She didn't even button her coat. She didn't notice the cold. She slipped and skidded through the slush. How easily she could be knocked over. My eyes sting when I see her rush off through a transformed city that now raised obstacles in her path.

She'd gone out into the world without a protective skin. You have to surround yourself with armour. You can't rely on the goodness of the world.

How could anyone be so cruel?

It wasn't cruelty, Mummy says.

What was it then? Daddy says.

I don't know, Mummy says. People have good intentions behind what they do.

She's always believed that cruelty comes with stabs and blows. That you can see it a long way off. That it marches forward in jackboots. She insists on believing that despite what she experienced.

Doubt rose inside her, it rose like water from beneath. It ran into her heart. How short it was, that feeling of liberation, a single happy walk through the winter city.

She crept deep into the office behind the shop. She sat there a long time, petrified with those words of judgment ringing in her ears. It was a judgment she had heard. You torment your child!

She threw herself over the table, buried her face in tissue paper and fabric. Was it a futile expedition out into the unknown with me, the spastic kid, the tormented victim? The other women, her colleagues, found her there. Let us help!

No, she wanted to be alone. They withdrew, frightened by the fierceness of her answer.

After an hour she began to telephone furiously. Now she had to ask those who could be asked. She had to get answers. Prepare herself against new attacks. That day and the following days she rang to specialists, she interviewed pediatricians. The sort of people who know, who should know.

She didn't talk to the Centre. She wanted it to be an independent investigation. She didn't talk to Daddy. It was her own investigation. She was searching for facts.

Facts! She introduced herself as a journalist. As a relative. As everything except what she was, the mother of a disabled child. The pediatricians she talked to were much as doctors usually are, careful, with a lot of on the one hand and a lot of on the other hand.

The doctor from Prague? Well, they themselves didn't have any experience of his method.

She squeezed it out of them. The doctor's method wasn't good.

How can you say that? Without any experience of your own.

We've heard from colleagues.

So you think there's no point in putting the children through the exercises?

One shouldn't express it quite so categorically.

But you don't recommend the Method?

One should think twice before using it.

You advise parents against it?

What did you say the name of the paper you work for is?

Click. I see the receiver sink down into the telephone. I see her hand holding it so tightly that her knuckles turn white.

She shouldn't have gone out into the world. She should have entrenched herself at home with her disabled kid, decorated her little idyll. Several times during her telephone calls she felt so sick she had to rush out to the toilet. She sank down over the WC and vomited.

Why didn't she stop questioning? She was burnt and yet she walked into the fire to be burned again.

The doctor from Prague is out of favour. His training programme is dropped.

It was the social welfare officer who said that. I don't know what sort of social welfare officer. She didn't belong to the Centre but must have had some connection with the physically disabled. It just says social welfare officer in the diary.

Mummy told the social welfare officer she could speak freely. Mummy'd got a new idea. She was preparing a newspaper article. She was reconnoitering, she said. That sounded professional. She'd heard the word on TV. As long as you are reconnoitering everyone could speak freely. They wouldn't be quoted.

The social welfare officer led Mummy into her office. The Authorities had furnished it with steel tubing and shining cupboards to dazzle the visitor. It was in Authority Bright style, Mummy says.

But the social welfare officer was human. She'd tried to make the room human. There were flowers in the windows. She'd hung pictures on the walls and replaced the official curtains.

How nice it is here, Mummy said. She felt sick. She pinched her leg to keep the feeling of sickness down.

The social welfare officer was a woman of about fifty with soft clothes of the kind children love to bury their noses in. She lay out friendly loops of words. So the doctor from Prague was being dropped. She wasn't in a position to assess it scientifically, but it was certainly a good thing that the Method was finally disappearing.

Why do you have such a poor opinion of it? Mummy asked.

It torments the children, the social welfare officer said.

Is that possible?

Unfortunately, she said. You don't know what the exercises consist of?

Mummy shook her head.

The children scream, the social welfare officer said.

But why . . . After all, the Method is still being used? Mummy spoke tonelessly, as though the words had lost their shape and their strength.

You see, at first we were happy about these new ideas, the social welfare officer said. We thought we were on the brink of a breakthrough. We didn't know that it was a matter of . . . Well, to be honest, something close to child abuse.

But if the children become better, Mummy said.

That's highly uncertain, the social welfare officer said. The medical experts are doubtful about it.

But all the same, suppose they become better?

At what cost? The social welfare officer began to analyze this. She lay out new and loving loops. She was a gardener who planted roses. We want to have secure children, happy children! Was it right that the poor spastic children should be torn apart, held down by parents they were bound to regard as bestial? She sighed. Her roses were edged with sorrow. She was a woman who takes suffering on herself, the suffering of defenceless children in the world.

Mummy dug her nails deeper into her leg. She listened and thought of the radio signals that wobble and fade and only get through in bursts from a remote transmitter.

The child's security must come first, the social welfare officer went on. Particularly during the first years. Everything indicates that. Children should be born gently, preferably at home, and not be guided or forced. They should start gently at the day nursery and at school. In fact, life itself should be welcomed so gently and so lightly that it almost isn't noticed. The social welfare officer talked about something she called a holistic view. One must have a holistic view of the child. She talked about the playful side of human beings, the delightful properties that are brought out in the child with the aid of love. Was it right then that disabled children should be tormented twice over, that they should be deprived of their infanthood?

We don't need more unhappy children, she said. She would never participate in a treatment that made children unhappy.

Mummy got up. She must have looked odd. It was as though a disease raged inside her and broke down the features of her face from within. A bloodstain spread over the pale fabric of her right trouser leg, just above the knee. She'd dug her nails in so hard her leg was bleeding. She hadn't noticed.

I lay on the table in front of her. That was what she saw. I lay there and blood rushed out of me.

Good heavens, the social welfare officer said. Oh, my dear!

Her first reaction was to keep it secret. No one was going to find out. The knowledge she had just gained was poisonous. She got it into her head that she had to protect Daddy. Protect what they were now doing.

She was going to hide her knowledge in a safe place. Steal out into the forest and find a hole and cover it with spruce twigs. As though new and even worse misfortunes threatened if he found out.

If only she could keep panic away.

How can such things be hidden? Daddy began to suspect that she was cheating with the exercises. He happened to come home earlier than expected. Was she finished already?

She managed to explain it away. She moved off. She wanted to sit alone. No, it was nothing in particular, she said. She just wanted to be by herself.

She could sit for hours by the children's beds. Berit was normal, she climbed and darted about like mad during the daytime. I wasn't normal. If there had been the slightest doubt about that, it was gone now. They'd been back to see the doctor with the French name.

I can see the result of their visit in the case records. Suddenly he detected lots of things wrong he hadn't noticed during the first visit. A whole catalogue of them. I was a basket case. Doesn't creep, it says. Doesn't sit. Doesn't roll. Stretched legs. Pointed foot.

He hadn't dared say it during the first visit. Mummy understood. Fear had obscured his vision. He had minimized the gravity of my illness. He didn't want to write a referral note to the Centre.

The Centre for tormenting misshapen children!

What sort of a game was going on? She hated the game because she was moved back and forth like a pawn. Most of all she hated herself for the thoughts she'd begun to think. Shouldn't they reduce the exercises? Tone them down?

You're destroying your child!

The words the social welfare officer had used struck her where she was most vulnerable. Of course she could work out a defence. They hadn't embarked on this unthinkingly. The social welfare officer gave her an unpleasant feeling. What use is it thinking when you've been hit at the heart of your emotions. Mummy felt dirty, covered with distrust.

How was she going to be able to say it to Daddy? We must break off the exercises. We've made a mistake. She didn't dare say it.

She could imagine fleeing. Sitting exactly like that beside our beds somewhere in a deserted house. Alone with us and the melancholic symphony of the wind.

I notice how my story is being pulled together. The cone of light is shrinking. I manipulate the spotlight. Mummy tries to run off. I capture her with the spotlight. Daddy stands in the centre of the stage with his big hands clenched in front of him. He's waiting for an opponent. He needs someone to knock down.

He invited people home. He wanted witnesses. He invited all sorts of people home, even remote acquaintances. They weren't going to put me through the exercises in secrecy. It was ridiculous to draw the curtains. The best thing would be to open the windows so that everyone knew.

Come round and see us! He invited the Rabble. They were going to have a jolly evening with wine and song. Like when they moved in.

Don't do it! Mummy tried to prevent it.

Why? He wondered about her. She who was so extrovert.

Not many people came. Didn't he notice how more and more were turning away from him? From us and from our house. But it was a relief that the composer kept away. He must have thought that our house was a disgusting place.

Those who came opened their eyes wide with surprise.

Elsa had asked to be there. She cooked the food and helped them with the preparations. Now she dressed in her nurse's uniform.

She looked radiant. The Rabble, who shambled around in worn jeans and flea-ridden manes of hair, almost had a fit when they saw her.

Daddy drank. He drank a lot. He laughed. Even at things you weren't supposed to laugh at. Vast silences occurred after his laughter. It was as though a signal system had broken down inside him and left him unable to see.

Mummy saw. Those who were there seemed embarrassed.

A man needs his friends, Daddy shouted, and raised his glass. The welcoming torches on the steps outside sent fire and flames across his face.

Now they were going to talk about cerebral palsy.

Let's sing, Mummy said.

We have nothing to hide, he objected. Have we?

He wanted to show them. But I was asleep. He wasn't the sort of man who wakes up his child in the middle of the night to show it off. He wasn't drunk.

He put down his glass on the table. That's the moment when I see him stand in the spotlight with his hands clenched in front of him.

Mummy shrank into herself. As though she hoped to disappear unnoticed.

Daddy told them about the children who'd been discovered twenty years ago. At that time there was no help. Some of them were operated on. Stretched muscles were cut off to make their limbs soft.

He told them about two English gymnasts who began to work with the children. In his album he's written Bobath. That was their name.

Three cheers for Bobath, an actor shouted.

No nonsense! Daddy raised his voice. He struck at the air with his clenched fist.

They really began to listen. He captivated his audience.

There was a violence in him, a desperation that they must have sensed.

He climbed up on a chair. He stood there, swaying above their heads. Up to now the children had been trained with positive stimulation.

Isn't that good?

All stimulation is good, Daddy roared and thumped the ceiling with his clenched fist. But they made a mistake, a decisive mistake.

Everyone fell silent. The audience was with him now.

Entice a spastic kid to creep! Of course, you can get the kid to creep across a floor. Across ten floors. But you're not getting at the injury. It's located here. He hit his hand against his head.

The injury is sitting there like a nail in the head. The kid can't use its legs the way normal kids do. When you get the kid to creep he must use a stick, an incorrect pattern of movement. And that reinforces the pathological state.

Daddy wrote the words in the air in front of them with letters a metre high. You wonder how I can know such things, things that should be beyond my understanding. But I know. They've told me. Again and again they've explained it. I could repeat it in my sleep. They wanted me to participate in what they were doing.

He must have talked for an hour at least. The glasses were empty. But they didn't notice. He led them on the way the doctor from Prague led them with his lantern. A major adventure!

Understand us. This is enormous. The doctor from Prague is a genius. Stop cracking and breaking the kids' legs. Stop enticing them deeper into their illness. Throw away the steel rails that have forced their feet into a right angle where no right angle existed.

The doctor's method is revolutionary!

Mummy didn't know where to hide. Listening was unbearable.

Everyone has started to use the Method now, Daddy said.

I can't imagine a more woeful scene. Why hadn't Mummy told him? The chair she sat on was a roller-coaster. She'd sat herself on it and now she was on her way down. Down into her own hell.

A triumph, Daddy said.

But isn't it painful for Asa? Their questions were eager.

She screams when she's doing the exercises, Daddy said. But in between she's happy.

All the same. Isn't it awful?

What's more awful? Sitting in a wheelchair all your life.

He carried them with him around this corner as well. Asa's getting a hell of a strong will, he shouted. She's a fighter. She'll be healthy. What is it the Chinaman says? Dig away the mountain, old man.

Asa will be healthy and she'll dig away ten mountains!

Mummy managed to get out of the room unnoticed. She fled into the kitchen and began to move the dishes around. The doctor from Prague is being dropped. That was the unequivocal answer her investigation had given. The method was useless.

She heard how they cheered and called out a toast.

§

What an evening! He sank down into the sofa when they'd gone, dazed by the wine and his victory. Listen! he called her. He needed her to share his triumph.

She blew out the candles.

Wasn't it fine?

Yes.

It was certainly a nice evening.

Yes.

She looked more and more like a shadow. She knew that his eyes were following her. She blew out the last candle. The flame vanished in a cloud of smoke. She's always so careful about using two wet fingers to extinguish the candles.Now she blew them out and candle grease flew over the table.

Everyone had fun, he said.

Yes.

They understand us and what we're doing with Asa.

Yes.

What's wrong then?

Is something wrong?

He asked her to sit beside him on the sofa. Come, let's sit a little while.

We're both sleepy, she said.

What's wrong with you?

I'm tired.

He got up so abruptly that several glasses were knocked over on the table in front of him. He rushed up to her. It was like an attack. He pulled her off with him to the sofa and pushed her down. Sit there!

I want to go to bed.

Now it was his turn to walk around the room. She should have said something. She closed her eyes, listened to his steps and knew that the disaster she'd waited for was on its way. No, she couldn't tell him. Particularly not now when he'd been drinking. She must protect him. Them. Something, whatever it was.

He followed the walls of the room. He'd found a track. He was like the old ogre in the fairytale who sniffs around in his cave and gets a whiff of Christian blood. I know that ogre. Daddy told us the fairytale when Berit and I were tiny tots.

The happy laughs had disappeared. Where did they go? They'd been dispersed like a flock of frightened birds. Daddy clenched his fist. It was as though the time of the clenched fists had come. They were like sledge hammers.

Cheating was what it was! He stood still. She cheated with the exercises.

No, she whispered.

Oh, he'd noticed all right. After the first suspicions he'd set up cunning traps.

If only she could sleep. Avoid this. He was spying on her. So what? Wasn't he right to do so? Her hands had begun to fumble. She'd begun to forget the movements. She wanted to forget them. How could she ever again put up with my cries of distress?

You have a bad conscience, Daddy rasped. Don't you think I saw you this evening. You kept out of the way. You felt ill. You're shirking and that's why things are going to hell.

No!

You skipped Asa's exercises today!

No.

I know you did.

Mummy couldn't imagine the disaster. She couldn't conceive of it in any other way than a sort of chaos of screams and blood. How his hands would begin to break things up, destroy, convert all the channels of agony to a single river of suffering.

At the last moment she found a secret door in the wallpaper, a means of escape she hadn't seen until then. With what remained of her strength she pushed open the door.

Asa has a temperature, she said.

She has a slight cold, Daddy said. That's no reason to skip the exercises.

Her temperature is higher, Mummy said.

I think she made it up. He was suspicious. But the moment of contact that makes the clouds shoot lightning over the ground stopped short. They went up to our room and there, right enough, I lay, red and hot, my breath panting.

Her temperature is far too high, Mummy said. We can't put her through the exercises.

Daddy collapsed into his bed.

Mummy moistened a towel and cooled my forehead. She took off my blanket and placed a thin sheet over me instead.

She felt unnatural. How can one be happy, almost happy because one's child has a temperature? She's told me about the temperature. I can look it up in the case history if I want to. I ended up in hospital for a few days. I was completely infected.

The temperature gave them a breathing space. They couldn't continue the exercises. Having a temperature can be so marvellous, so wonderfully pleasant!

§

Her happiness was short-lived.

I'm lying on the examination bed again. They're standing around the bed. I can see them like small dolls. My story reduces them. I put them in front of me on the desk now that morning is pressing its nose against my window.

Aunt Tilly usually says that small people have small problems. The dolls look silly. It's best to have them small and reduced. All frightening stories should begin like that. I put the rabbit in the waste paper basket. She doesn't like sitting there. But I don't think the end of my story would be good for her. She's so sensitive.

I scream and kick about.

I do what I can to translate my screams. Although I've always heard a lot about the exercises, most of it has been vague. At first I didn't bother so much about it. Not even when they shouted "spastic" after me at school.

Even then I didn't bother so much about it. I felt hurt, of course. But that passed. Now I know I must go back. Into myself and them, as we were then.

It's as though I'd need to give a terrific yell to really get rid of it. Bawl like that time so that I'll get enough force to open the window when the light comes, and sneeze at the first beams of sunlight. I and my rabbit.

They're at the Centre. Mummy stands there with at least a hundred questions but she can get out almost nothing.

The physical therapist points and examines. During

the time when I had a temperature I've deteriorated. I'm more tense. Above all there's something wrong with my eyes.

Daddy bends forwards. I wave my arms. Pick me up! Help me get out of here!

He lets me lie. He looks at my eyes. They're less steady now, much less steady than two weeks ago.

The physical therapist sends out her abrupt messages. Now we know. She gets worse when you don't do the exercises with her.

And better when we do the exercises with her . . . Daddy says it. He sinks down and remains sitting on the floor. He's trying to understand this remarkable connection. We do exercises with her legs, he says slowly and then her gaze becomes steadier.

Good God! Can anyone understand it? This is the fantastic journey out into the Milky Way he'd been hoping for. The journey he'd believed so much in.

Mummy looks as well. How can she present her doubts now? This means more exercises. A new thread to hold on to. But how strong is it? How strong are they?

Don't make me go through it!

The world is divided into soft and hard. My tiny body clutches what's soft. What's good. Mummy's talked to the social welfare officer. The warm and kind social welfare officer wants to leave the children alone.

Mummy's talked to the pediatricians. If there was any good in the world the social welfare officer and the pediatricians would help me now. Save me.

That's what my cries mean.

One can lie in peace in the soft hiding spots of the world. Spastic kids aren't trained against their will there.

I shout for Granny. The dolls in front of me turn their heads to see who I'm shouting for. Granny is outside their circle. She's sitting a little further away on my pen-case. She's my last hope.

Why don't you save me?

You must put your trust in your parents, she says.

But they're out of their minds.

They're wiser than you are.

They've sold themselves and me to the hard world.

You must do your exercises, you must break through, you must fight.

I don't want to.

You can!

I want to be what I am. To lie as I lie. Quiet, motionless. It doesn't matter that I'll be twisted. I shan't annoy anyone. I'll lie like a small, injured kitten in a corner without making any trouble. Why doesn't Mummy listen to the warm, kind people?

Your Mummy is kind.

I scream. Things will turn out badly for me.

Not at all, Granny says.

She's still sitting on the edge of the pen-case. She's so well-dressed and elegant. I've never heard her become angry or raise her voice. But I know how she can sound when she's decided on something. Uncompromising. Without the slightest sign of doubt. Now she's talking with her uncompromising voice. It won't turn out badly for Asa. That's a lie. Admittedly she screams. But she's also becoming better.

Between the exercises you're much happier now, she says.

I'm not going to listen to you, I say. I thought you were on my side.

She talks about those who freeze to death. They say it's a pleasant feeling to freeze. You lie in the snow and feel warm. The most pleasant moment of all comes just when you're about to die.

That's exactly how I want to lie, I say. The way the people who are soft and warm want children to lie. Why can't they leave me in peace?

Nonsense, she says and walks away.

I hate her. My screams say that I hate her and what they're doing to me.

Of course, they're not really like that! My parents aren't like that at all. By now you ought to know what they're like. They were like butterflies in a grey forest. Until I was born.

They pull up a mass of principles out of a gloomy well. But the principles don't suit them. Mummy dreams of putting on her false eyelashes again. Of becoming as she was before.

She's dreaming of the time she danced on the headmaster's desk. She was fifteen then, she wore a brace on her teeth and danced naked on the headmaster's desk.

I hear her protest. It wasn't on the headmaster's desk.

What desk was it on?

It was on the desk in the teacher's common-room, she says and giggles.

That's what she's like really! She dreams about her trousers. When she went to school she'd dyed one leg of her trousers red and the other green. Then she began to become infatuated with the Chinese. I think it's the same infatuation. There's no other explanation for why she still has a green tuft in her red hair.

She's a dreamer, just like Daddy. I know that he was wild and carefree. He played music at dances when he was a teenager. He still has his trumpet, it's hanging on the wall. He played hooky from school. He learnt to imitate Aunt Tilly's handwriting, he forged excuses and skipped school. He got a C for conduct.

That part of him that Mummy calls his ordinariness paranoia, trying to be like everyone else . . . It's all on the surface. It's not really him.

They're dreamers. When they met life was one big celebration. They hadn't the slightest thought of becoming adults. Now everything has changed—because of me.

§

Leave me alone! Don't make me do the exercises!

My screams should move them. They're not made for digging out mountains with a shovel. They'll never manage it.

But on this day, as I lie on the examination bed and they look at my unsteady eyes, they decide to continue.

Chapter Eleven

The weeks passed and winter had now been overcome. The city awoke each morning in the bright costume of early spring. Just thinking of it is enough to make one smile.

The snow became wet and shiny. Melted snow dripped from the roofs, and the thin ice covering the pools of water on the street crackled in the mornings.

The warm little corner at the front of the house was already clear of snow. We could lie there and take an afternoon nap while Elsa was busy in the kitchen and everything white in the world shone in through the windows.

Our little house had tricked the storms, had cheated destiny and had survived another roaring winter. A few planks had come loose. A gutter hung down crookedly. It was no worse than that.

A gingerbread house! That's how I see it. A gingerbread house without a witch. They had no need for a witch there, they could have followed Mummy's impulse and hidden themselves in the innermost parts of the house with their fantasies and their misfortune, hidden themselves with me, their spastic kid. They could have taken time off from their work, they could have cleaned out Aunt Tilly's dog-eared bank-book and only done what was absolutely necessary—put me through my exercises, taken care of the other children and themselves.

They needed time. They thought it was I who demanded their time. But they were wrong. They needed time for themselves.

Mummy could have stayed at home and dreamt about

her promised land where the sun rises, about the fat Chinaman and about the sources from which the world's justice is said to flow out.

Daddy wanted to write poems. He could have sat there the way they'd thought he would when first they saw the house, at the window in what's now my room, and let the glittering snow and the clouds decide his thoughts.

They could have sat down a while, rested themselves.

Granny told me a story once. It's a story from Africa, from the time when there were still bearers. One day, after marching for many miles, the bearers suddenly sat down. We refuse to go a step further, they said. We're stopping to give our spirits time to catch up with us.

How are we to look into the future? How are we to know that spirits of a completely different kind sweep in when you happen to leave the door open?

I see them rush off, always in a hurry. Everything around them became increasing confusion. Everything except my exercises. They'd devoted themselves to cutting their moorings without noticing the malignant spirits that were after them all the time.

They put me through my exercises and my eyes became a little steadier again. They concentrated themselves on the task even more, if that were possible. They also thought they could see my free leg begin to bend, the leg that was not locked in position during the exercises. First the right-hand leg and then the left-hand leg.

Daddy clung to these small advances as though they were of great value. He examined them over and over again. He had found the hidden treasure and he went to it to regard each new jewel.

Their bodies rolled and wound themselves around mine on the little table where the gym mat lay. They were as naked as I was, as vulnerable and unprotected as I was. The weight of their bodies was enormous and yet their care transformed their weight to feathers and air.

Except the part that locked me in position, the part that

was to make me, to make my will break through the damage in my brain.

They still had evenings when they talked. But they had more and more difficulty in finding the stillness that conversation requires. You have to find a length of shore, that's how I see it, a length of shore with shining water, whirling mosquitos and a warm jetty to sit on. A place where your spirit can catch up with you and where you take time to listen and to understand.

Mummy said something about her investigation. That there were those who had doubts about the Method.

Of course, he said. Not everyone can have the same opinion.

A lot of doubt, she said. More and more people are abandoning it.

The telephone rang. It always rang, it shrilled and blared when they were going to talk. Or else it was the washing up or the cleaning up or the tiredness of each evening that seemed to grow heavy as lead.

The physical therapist talked more openly now. There were different opinions. But they shouldn't bother about that.

Asa'll get better, Daddy said. Now we can see it.

Just the same. Mummy tried to reach him.

You're a Cassandra, Daddy said. No matter what people say, we have science on our side.

He didn't want to listen. Mummy had experienced his violence, a dark portent of a coming disaster. It was like walking around with a taste of blood in your mouth. For him everything depended on the tiny improvement they saw in me. Everything!

We must protect what we're fond of. It's when I creep down into her bed that she returns to that. She thinks of the pensive moments on the lake shore. Hard words are like stones. They hide things but they don't provide strength. Look at the moon! It shines, but without heat.

The words that give strength are small, lost words, intimate words of love. That's what's wonderful and odd.

If only they'd had a moment like that together!

But they were caught up in their own hurry. They created hurry. Their hands needed a thousand things to do so they wouldn't have to think so much.

I see a growing confusion, but also how small laughs get in their way. It seems melancholy. Like watching their last chance, the last chance for them and for our home.

I see Mummy attend parents' day. Conscientious parents visit their children's schools. Now it was parents' day in Lisa's class.

Mummy didn't have time. But of course she wanted to go for Lisa's sake. Inside her she was exploding with the thought of all the things parents should participate in. During the short walk to the school she'd thought bloodthirsty thoughts about the Lucia Day celebrations her neighbour had had to go through recently.

Her neighbour had four children, one of whom went to a day nursery, another to the kindergarten and the other two to different schools. It began with the morning celebrations of Lucia Day on TV. Then, of course, there were the Lucia celebrations in the schools and at the other institutions. In the evening the swimming club had a Lucia Day swim and the scouts arranged a torch-lit procession to the church. All in all, Mummy's neighbour went through about ten Lucia Day celebrations and ended up with an aching stomach.

We should have one point seven children, Daddy says. Neither more nor less. That's the average.

Now Mummy sat in the classroom. She sat along the wall beside the respectable mothers, the one point seven mothers. It was Monday and the teacher wanted to know what the children had done during the weekend.

Everyone put up their hand. The teacher selected Kalle.

Kalle began to tell them. First of all his Daddy had made a lot of telephone calls. Then they drove off in the car. The whole family.

And where did you drive to? the teacher asked.

She smiled. Kalle was a lively storyteller. The one point seven mothers also smiled. The only one who didn't smile was Kalle's Mummy. She looked as if she'd got a venemous insect inside the back of her dress.

We drove for mile after mile, Kalle said. To buy the equipment.

What equipment? the teacher asked.

The home-distilling equipment, Kalle said.

I see, the teacher said and didn't know what to say. Kalle had time to tell everyone about the tubes and hoses and about the Sunday evening experiments in the basement, while the silence grew more and more deafening, before the teacher got around to thanking him for his account.

Mummy laughed that evening. Life offered them its moments. Don't run away from laughter! That forms part of those days. Laughter rings out and fades. Ridicule dies away. There are moments. Make use of them!

Like the story about Elsa. Another story about forbidden bottles. That's the way it is, Daddy says. Can I help it?

Elsa rang Daddy at work. It was in the middle of an important conference.

Hello, Elsa called. You must come.

What's up? Daddy said. Inside him he saw his home go up in flames.

I've been arrested, Elsa whimpered in her broadest SmÅland accent. I'm at the Åland ferryboat. Putte bit someone and I've been arrested. You must come.

I don't have time, Daddy said. What happened?

You must come!

Daddy threw himself into a taxi. He'd heard Elsa's need and couldn't just leave her in the lurch.

When he arrived at the Åland ferryboat he found there was a great fuss at the customs. Elsa stood in the middle of it all. By turns she cried and cursed a whole bunch of uniformed customs officers.

Elsa had bottles in her bag. She'd put Putte on top of the

bag. She wasn't going to let the customs men search through it. When a customs officer tried to he was bitten.

Putte was in his angriest mood. So was the customs officer who'd been bitten.

I can have you prosecuted for this, the customs officer said.

My God, Elsa sobbed, I'm sick. I'm going blind. It's your fault. If you touch me I'll die.

There must be a misunderstanding, Daddy said.

Like hell there's a misunderstanding, the customs officer snapped and dried blood from his hand with a handkerchief.

This lady is religious, Daddy said. She's a member of the Pentacostal Movement and would never dream of smuggling.

She claimed she didn't have anything to declare, the customs officer said.

She's hard of hearing, Daddy said.

She's hard of hearing and she's going blind, the customs officer said. Ha ha ha!

Yes, Daddy shouted. There are actually people who neither hear nor see well. I can vouch for her. You shouldn't persecute people who are old and sick. Things like that can get in the papers.

He managed to pick up the growling Putte by the neck without being bitten, to lift out a couple of bottles from Elsa's bag and slam them down on the counter, and make off with her in a taxi.

Thanks, Elsa sighed when they were sitting in the taxi.

That was a silly thing to do, Daddy said.

You've no idea how wicked they were to me, Elsa said.

She began to search with one hand inside her dress. Daddy stared at her. She fished out a bottle from one of the hiding places in her body. Here, she said, it's for you. You're so awfully kind.

Mummy laughed. They sat around the table in the kitchen. Elsa'd gone home. Berit sat at one end of the table in her baby chair. Mummy held me in her arms. What a story! It's simply too funny!

I'll break that mongrel's neck, Daddy said.

What? At first they couldn't believe their ears.

Didn't you hear me? I'm going to kill that beast!

He meant it. They left the table without finishing their food. Daddy sat on alone. The time for laughing was over. The merriment faded away. Our home faded away.

The days grew longer. The exercises ground on drearily and the first hopes began to fade. The worst of all was that I was screaming more. Hair-raising screams! Every fibre in my body screeched for an end to what they were doing.

Mummy and Daddy worked in shifts. They met each other in the doorway. They hugged each other quickly and quickly exchanged a few words. Then they stopped hugging each other. At night they slept back to back. They forgot to say goodnight.

They blamed it on the lack of time. Being short of time became an excuse. As though a friendly smile takes time! As though they only had a tiny hole left in their hearts and that hole was filled with me, the spastic kid who had to be put through her exercises.

And I showed no noticeable improvement.

Mummy was absent-minded. She put things down and she couldn't remember where she'd put them. Daddy tripped over things left lying about on the stairs and on the floor.

As usual, he was the first to get up in the mornings. He laid the breakfast table for Lisa, Patrick and himself. He prepared baby rice for us infants. Ever since they met he's always given Mummy coffee in bed. He usually says it was his big mistake. When they met and fell in love he made the mistake of signing a contract about coffee in bed.

Just imagine! Spouting out a thing like that!

Now she didn't want to wake up. She didn't want any coffee. She held on to her pillow and her sleep as though the new day threatened to be worse than any other day.

He grew surly. His tone became sharper. He claimed she wanted to spend all day in bed, eating chocolates.

Patrick was impossible to wake. Daddy's attempts grew into a sort of ritual that always ended up with a row. Daddy's noted it in his diary, the beginning of the eternal morning rows.

He began by calling gently: Breakfast is ready! He called twice. A little louder the second time. The third time he shouted. Then he got bawled out.

Bloody hell! Patrick shouted. What are you shouting at me for? Why didn't you wake me earlier?

Patrick didn't have time to eat breakfast.

There I was with my nicely laid breakfast table, Daddy says. No one wanted to wake up.

Of course no one wanted to wake up, Mummy says. You were always in such a bad humour.

Even today they can't talk about the morning in their lives when the black rows were born. The playful pushing and butting didn't apply anymore. Suddenly it was serious.

It's so ridiculous. My parents can be the most ridiculous people alive. How could they begin to quarrel about petty things? I hate their quarrels. I'd be willing to hurt myself, to cut myself in the arm, if it would make them stop.

Daddy had been a little more gentle and kind for a while. Now he grew tense again. My body and my lack of progress acted as a barometer for his black moods.

He used the breakfast table as a punishment for those who were ungrateful. Laying it became a sort of revenge. Mummy scarcely touched the coffee he put beside her bed. She simply disappeared out through the front door like a blue wreath of smoke.

You must put away the things you've left on the stairs, he said as she went.

I'll do it, she said. Oh, what a lot of nagging!

They've been lying there for a week now! He stood in the front door and shouted out across the street so that the neighbours heard.

That was what it was like when they said good morning to each other. Our home faded away, our happy and lovely little home.

They weakened themselves and began to seek out faults in each other. Anyone who makes an effort can always find faults. Evil spirits crossed the threshold with a whole load of silliness. Who's cut the bread without wiping away the crumbs after them? Why is there no towel in the lavatory?

Because I put it with the dirty laundry.

Why didn't you hang out a new one?

Can you imagine adults quarrelling about things like that! Is that what growing up involves?

I'd like to stop my story and call to them down through the years. Have you forgotten your purpose? The world is perishing. You know that. My world and your world is breaking up, and you quarrel about towels and bread-crumbs!

You let yourselves be led out into an adventure. You used the word yourselves. You put your faith in a doctor from Prague, a friendly little man who made Jesus's cause his own.

That was the way you saw it. You were going to take me, an injured and unhappy child, in your hands and wander out into the darkness. Brave the dangers! You were going to make me healthy. But there was more to it than that. You wanted to prove something.

Have you forgotten? You're destroying my story with your wretched drivel about breadcrumbs and coffee in the mornings. You had a nobler purpose. What was it you said?

I search through the photos in front of me on the desk. Here it is! This was the photo you saved, the young people on the truck. The flag opens out, the flag of freedom. Let me remind you of your own words, that you now seem to have forgotten. The iron-hard caterpillers crawled over the city of Prague. Evil spat out the dream of a new world. Evil spat as though it had a worm in its mouth. It can't stand freedom.

I was the child that was born, the mangled child.

The doctor from Prague found a refuge in your hearts. You gave him room in the way you've always given room to refugees. The child can be made healthy. The dream is not in vain. The world can be made healthy. Those are your words!

The adventure didn't turn out the way you thought it would. You longed for glittering sunshine and winter streets. Instead you got the hopeless, murderous routine of exercises, schedules and discipline. You weren't prepared for it. When you were most in need of simple, kind words you tore them out of your lives. You tore them out the way children strip the Christmas tree of its decorations. You threw everything into a container, the sort of container Aunt Tilly pokes around in once it's dark.

My rabbit is scratching about in the wastepaper basket where I've put her. I stretch down my hand and caress her soft fur. No matter how I try I can't change my story.

Mummy longed to get away. Her duties at home became heavier and heavier. She did what she was supposed to do. She put me through the exercises when she was supposed to do it, she wrote excuses for Patrick, she shopped at the Co-op, and accomplished everything that was supposed to be accomplished. She did her duty, but nothing more.

And when she was at work she longed to go home. She wanted to be at home and feed us, to put things right and to carry her little ones around the way cats carry their squealing kittens by the nape of the neck. She would have spent more time at home if it hadn't been for Daddy. He was always quarrelling.

They were exhausted. They looked ahead and saw nothing except new and even drearier days. It makes me think of poor quality chinaware. A little knock and it cracks.

Science supports us, supports what we're doing with Asa. Daddy repeated these words and made them sound like a magic formula. He talked about Science as though there was some kind of Council of Enlightenment, a dwelling for wise men with all the wisdom of the world collected in their silver-haired heads.

When he did my exercises with me he called out to the dumb walls to convince them. Science is truth and life. We don't have to bother about a few petty pediatricians who doubt. Listen to me, Asa! The pediatricians don't understand what we're doing. They poke about in nasal catarrh and prescribe penicillin. They're as smart as a bunch of bicycle repairmen who've been retrained as veterinary surgeons.

Fight, Asa, fight!

I kicked with my leg. I clutched the red stick. I screamed.

Bend your leg!

He felt the impotence of despair. My will wasn't enough. He felt the impotence as a creeping temptation within him. The temptation to take my legs in his strong hands, to break them straight, to break my body the way nature didn't want it to be.

No! He let go of me and sank down on the gym mat. We're doing what's right because Science says so. Don't cry, old girl. We'll make it.

He crept down from the table, and took me in his arms.

I can see him sitting there in the sofa, his arms about me. He presses me against his naked chest. I'm crying and I think that he's crying. I've never seen him cry but I know he did it sometimes when we were going through the exercises.

§

That photo! I can't get away from that photo. Daddy alone with me, muttering his formulas. Mummy's more shadowy now, with comforting words that grow weaker and weaker.

They sought moments when they could be alone. Being together caused them anguish. They wanted to put me through the exercises without being observed. As though at any moment they risked being caught cheating or crying or showing some other weakness. But solitude didn't give them strength. Just more anguish.

A tiny little push and they'd fall. Daddy had his new straw to clutch, the straw he called Science, the society of the silver-haired. Now Science came to him. He was alone that evening. The children were asleep. He lit a fire in the tiled stove. The March sky lay like a crystal bowl above the city. I can see our house, how the light shines from the windows in the big room, and I can see Daddy's silhouette inside as he sits at the desk.

He'd heard about a magazine. If you want to know what Science says, read this!

It was a magazine for physical therapists. He's saved it amongst all the other documents. I can read it just as he read it that evening. A senior physician expressed his opinion, one of the famous, a specialist in spastic children at the big hospital on the north side of the city.

Daddy riffled through the magazine. He found the article. I can see his hands hold the magazine and his body, a little round-shouldered, bend over it.

Science came into the open and talked. The content was as clear as the sky above the roof of the house.

There are no scientific facts behind what you're doing.

Daddy stared.

It's an open question if you're not further disabling a child who is already disabled, the doctor went on.

What's he saying? Daddy read the first paragraphs again.

The fire crackled in the stove. The black letters freed themselves from the pages and became a voice and a face. Science stood in front of Daddy and spoke with cold assurance.

Daddy moved back so violently the chair almost tipped over. He let go of the magazine and held onto the armrests.

The doctor from Prague has no theoretical basis for his activities, the senior physician wrote.

It can't be true!

You don't believe me?

No!

You wanted to talk to Science. Wasn't that it? You got a warning. But you didn't listen to the warning your wife gave you.

A sharp crack came from the stove. Embers shot out over the floor. Daddy didn't notice them.

You chose to be blind. It wasn't science you sought. It was faith. The doctor from Prague is guessing. His guesses are arbitrary and absurd.

In exactly the same way Mummy had sat and listened when the social welfare officer closed off the cracks in a wall in front of her. But it was worse now. The cell was completely walled in. Now it was Science that had closed the door and turned the key.

Was there no benefit at all in the exercises then?

There's a risk of fractures, the senior physician wrote. A risk that you may injure your child.

But nothing at all?

The only palpable results are the negative side effects.

We're not injuring her!

The senior physician paused a moment, as though Daddy's protests would die off through their own inherent weakness. What argument could Daddy put up when Science spoke? Look for yourself, you foolish man, look before the last light is extinguished. Asa isn't getting any better. You claim you've seen a few almost unnoticeable changes. Her eyes, yes! But that's nothing.

People with authority fixations are attracted by a tough, no-nonsense approach. They want cures that meet this criteria. This is their simple and meaningless recipe.

Daddy got up. He could have sworn the senior physician had been standing right there in the room talking to him. Now there was no one there. He bent down in front of the stove and closed the little doors. The embers had left black marks on the floor.

The crystal bowl darkened above our house.

He picked up the magazine and read it again. There the article was, in print, and it wasn't a dream.

§

Again I see the photo, the photo Daddy kept secret. How the tears gleam on his cheeks and how he presses me to his naked chest. Don't cry, Asa!

Men don't cry, particularly not a Daddy who's big and strong. It's only at the cinema they cry sometimes.

But this wasn't the cinema and it wasn't a dream. He sat in the theater office. The show-down they'd been preparing for months was in progress all around him. But it was as though it had long since ceased to concern him.

He had two lives now. The lightning had finished splitting him. He was there amongst them, at work, and yet it was with me he sat. It was me he held in his arms.

They said they didn't get on well with Daddy. They wanted to discuss his manner, his ways.

Don't cry, Asa! Let's not listen to them. We'll find a way of being happy again. I know how to make people laugh.

You're so cold, an actor said.

What? Daddy asked. The voices around him were like a swarm of mosquitos. What are you saying?

I think you're cold as ice, the composer said.

And hard!

They'd made a list of his bad points. He was unkind and sarcastic. He made fun of people.

He heard himself answer. But it was only half of him. They couldn't know that he sat with me in his arms. I'll hide you close to me, Asa. Death knocked at our door. Let's hug each other and ignore it.

What you lack is warmth, they went on.

Do I have to hold your hands? he said.

You're authoritarian, they said.

Prepare a room for me in the cellar, he said. Lock me in there. Send in food through a little opening.

He refused to apologize. Those who have talked with death don't grovel before others. He was like an old farmer who finally takes down his gun from the wall to defend what he's built. He'd prefer to put the house on fire than let them in. He'd prefer that.

They thought he was too tough. They wanted him to be softer.

He grew furious. He whispered to me. Lie here quietly, Asa. I'm just going to kill a few of them. They're snakes, soft snakes that attack from the rear.

He didn't want to be soft. He was a professional, he said. He'd worked for newspapers. Who the hell asks for softness. He'd written the plays for the theatre. With those plays he'd helped workers who had dust in their lungs, he'd helped lumberjacks who became sick from sawing.

Hundreds of thousands of people had seen his plays. The theater had become famous. The actors had their pictures in the gossip magazines and could drink sweet wine every day. All because of what Daddy had written for them.

He had neither time nor desire to be soft. If any of them wanted a nanny he could always go home and fuck his mother.

He came out with the most awful things he could think of. He was like an arsonist. Once again he held me in his arms and his secret tears made his cheeks gleam. Science had said what it had to say. Death had breathed on our home. The enemy was already inside but they wouldn't take him alive, neither him nor me.

That confirms it, an actor said.

You're harder than we thought, the composer said.

They called in two specialists. Daddy calls them family therapists. They usually arrange courses, quarrel courses, for people who quarrel a lot. Now they were going to make Daddy kinder, but in fact they had the opposite effect. If they thought they could scratch about in his soul, they were mistaken. He had no intention of letting himself be opened. He wasn't canned goods.

People like my plays, he said.

Well, about his plays. It was his plays that were the problem. They'd finally got to what it was all about. Digging around in Daddy's entrails had only been a preparation.

How were they going to get rid of him?

The whole theater sat down for a mass meeting. Daddy had made a fool of himself. He'd frightened off his friends and got his enemies to sharpen their teeth. The mass meeting took several weeks. Everyone wanted to decide. There's nothing worse, Daddy says.

All the time Daddy sat there with me. He and I were invisible to the world and to them. Don't cry, Asa, see how cheerfully the fire crackles when I light it.

You write clumsily, they told him.

So coarsely!

You think the workers are too coarse? he taunted them.

We want plays with more soul in them. When you get down to it, the workers have souls as well.

So you've discovered that the workers have souls, Daddy said.

Of course the workers have souls, a pimply dentist's son, who'd played the worker hero in several plays, said.

Can you prove it? Daddy grinned. He suggested that they write an article with the heading: Do workers have souls?

He became more and more unbearable. They thought he was disgusting.

We want to act in proper plays, they said.

You want bigger pictures in the gossip magazines, Daddy said.

God how they must have detested him. The mass meetings took weeks. They couldn't decide. They decided one thing one day and tore it up the next. When they couldn't decide on the big things they devoted themselves to the small. It must have been dreadful. Several of the actors had nervous breakdowns and fearful scenes took place.

It took them three days to decide the colour of a false nose. One of the actors rushed over to the window.

It must be red, he shouted. If you can't decide I'm going to throw myself out.

He was already sitting with his legs over the window frame when they managed to pull him in.

The false nose was red. It was the only decision they managed to reach during two weeks.

I see Daddy stand up one day, with the look of someone who has finally reached a decision. He'd hoped they'd fire him. But they were too cowardly, he says. They didn't have the courage even for that.

Daddy stands there. His self-destructive day of work is over. He holds me pressed against his heart. Not for a single second during these days has he let me go. He looks mean and wicked. I feel sorry for him. But I don't understand his dark desire to destroy.

He places his new play on the table. Do what you like with it, he says and walks out. He's gone before they have time to react, he's off with his spastic kid to see if there's anything left to smash.

Chapter Twelve

This happened in March. Days of decision.

I see Mummy search for a key. She's got a key hidden. Only she knows where it is. I'm with her. Just like Daddy, whe holds me, struggles with me, caresses me.

She finds the key and steals in through a door that's just for her and me. She's a dream person. On the other side of the door her wonderland opens up. I can see her happy face and her eyes shining at what they see.

This is the country that never ends. This is the country where the sun rises and where you can sit beside the springs. This is where the springs of justice, that she so often talks about, flow out.

She walks there with me, her child, pressed against her body. People are working and singing everywhere. People welcome you wherever you go. People welcome me, the spastic kid!

Everything is possible in Wonderland. This is where they dig out mountains. A hundred thousand men and women, dressed in blue, dig and sing and play bamboo flutes.

The fat Chinaman with the wart is sitting in the centre of Wonderland. He raises his hand and blesses his people. The great oarsman, he's called.

Now flowers rain down and colourful children dance along the roads. Do you know, Asa, Mummy says . . . Do you know that the only structure the first astronauts on the moon saw was the Great Wall.

She carries me in under an apricot tree. We sit in the cool shade and listen to the water which runs in the canals.

Of course it was a dream. She'd be angry if she heard me tell it. She's not naive. Not as naive as that. Although I think she understood then that, basically, it was the same dream as the dream the doctor from Prague carried with him on his long flight. He saw the child and the shepherds. Mummy saw the shining fish that glittered in the pond beyond the old pagoda.

Of course she knew that sorrows and troubles exist there. As they do everywhere. But hope, that was real amongst the dancing children in the rain of flowers. What man can do. The dragons can be conquered. Have you seen the Chinese monkey on television, the monkey in the old Chinese story, the monkey that went with the monk to India over a thousand years ago, the monkey that plays with the black dragons in the clouds?

There's hope for the tiniest beings in the world. For you and me, Asa! For us. You're going to become like the king who plays with the dragons. You're going to become healthy.

That was her dream and now she needed it more than ever on that evening in March when she met the Chinese. I don't think she'd ever met any Chinese before. Now she stood amongst real Chinese, eager and curious.

Someone in our district had invited the staff of the Chinese embassy home. Mummy was also invited. With me present and hidden, as usual, inside her, she searched for someone to talk to. I can imagine how she longed to find confirmation. How she wanted dream and reality to be united.

After the meal people moved around and she found a young Chinawoman. What about spastic children in China? How are they treated?

The Chinawoman looked at her blankly. Mummy had to repeat her question.

Oh, you mean disabled children, the Chinawoman said. There aren't any in China.

Mummy looked into two eyes black as coal.

There aren't any, the Chinawoman repeated.

I don't understand, Mummy said.

We have Socialism in China, the Chinawoman said. There are no disabled children under Socialism.

I don't believe that.

Well, that's the way it is, there aren't any.

Mummy left. She sat on a bench in the park. Almost all the snow had gone, except on the northern slopes.

What if you'd been born in China, Asa?

She doesn't exist.

What if you'd been born there and we discovered you were disabled?

Doesn't exist.

A dream is torn apart. It can be like dying, only worse. She saw pictures of horror rush out under the desolate park lamps. What does one do with people who don't exist?

She'd heard it before. She thought of the railway wagons that were emptied of their human contents. She felt the smell of smoke prickle in her nose. We remove the crippled, the disabled, the ill. They've been condemned from life. There's no room for them.

It couldn't be true. She must have met someone crazy. Even amongst the Chinese there must be people who lack judgment. But the woman she met wasn't crazy, she knew it in the depth of her consciousness. The Chinawoman was a young, talented diplomat, employed at the Chinese embassy.

When the dream crashes in smithereens, obvious and ingrained words get a new meaning. Mummy tried them with a desperate melancholy.

Those who don't work won't eat! That's what they had said. She'd said it herself. The Socialists said it.

You can't work, Asa. You're disabled, so you won't be allowed to eat.

Those who till the soil shall be entitled to it. She'd applauded when she heard that. I see it in her diary. She'd been to the theatre and seen a play by someone called Brecht. A German.

You'll never be entitled to the soil, Asa. And you won't be allowed to eat.

She sat for a long time on the park bench. Not until she was so cold she shivered did she walk home. There was nothing, no dream, no happiness. There was only me.

§

And Daddy.

They couldn't talk to each other any longer. He rushed around the house with the eyes of Science staring at his back.

They couldn't make peace in our little nest. They didn't have enough force to protect their young. The world outside broke up their hiding place and pushed them out on icy expanses where there was no shelter in sight.

What you're doing is meaningless! When Daddy heard the judgment of Science it was as though he decided to complete what was meaningless down to the last sigh of the disaster.

He blew up. But I don't know if it was his fault alone. Mummy is so clever when she quarrels. She quarrels with the aid of silence. I know she can drive him mad with silence.

I hear their crying and their shouts. They sort out everything ridiculous and made it a reason for quarrelling. I see the nest broken apart and how the snake waits outside with cold eyes. Even when the danger became clear they still fought each other, almost drunk with grief.

Old Elsa withdrew. She had enough suffering of her own. You can't stand cooking sprat-and-potato pie when the house is being attacked by demons.

They could have asked for help from the quarrel experts. Absorbed by the breakdowns described in their diaries, I notice how giggly I become. It doesn't seem right. I giggle despite how awful it is. I think of the quarrel experts' attempts with Daddy. Quarrels must be carried through with style. I know. I've read a lot about quarrels. A quarrel should be organized like you organize an essay in school. First you make your layout, with the introduction, conflict and climax, finished off with an artistic finale. Then you start your quarrel.

If you're the best in the class you get five out of five. Quarrels should be elegant.

Their quarrels were ugly and coarse. They were the worst in the class. I think they wanted to be. Those who are worst in the class spit and kick.

Mummy stayed silent until she got Daddy to explode, since that was her unfailing method. The house collapsed. Daddy tried to remain silent too but couldn't. He said wicked things.

There you are! She was constantly presented with new proofs of how nasty he was.

She got him off balance. But in fact he was off balance all the time. He began to throw things around. That was further proof of his nastiness.

They said things. You're like your mother. It was Daddy who said it first. Just like your mother! I don't understand it. I don't understand how adults think. I don't understand how that's the worst thing they can find to say. You're like your mother.

In the evenings Daddy stood at the window and waited for Mummy. She was late. She didn't telephone. He lay the table beautifully and lit the candles. He knew she was avoiding coming home. Anguish hung in the room like a sour smell.

She stayed away longer and longer. He thought she had someone else. I don't dare consider it. When she finally came home the candles had burnt out. They quarrelled all night.

Daddy picked on Patrick when Mummy was away. He chased after Patrick. Patrick had to learn to give a hand.

Daddy tried to educate Patrick. He read him the tale about Casper who didn't eat his soup. When Patrick heard the tale he never ate soup again.

Patrick became more cheeky. He shouted out four-letter words. He had no intention of giving a hand. The end came closer. One morning rage ran riot.

Daddy struck Patrick.

Mummy rushed out. She took her children, Lisa and Patrick, and went off with them to the sofa in the livingroom. She held her arms about them.

He must learn, Daddy shouted and shook his fists above their heads.

Don't listen to him, Mummy whispered.

Daddy lifted a chair and threw it on the ground. Now they were forced to listen. His rage was a terminal point. He blamed Mummy. It was Mummy who had made him wicked. She and her kids!

His rage was mixed with scorn. Mummy neglected her children. She devoted her evenings to other things. But now she had the chance to play at being a good mother. What play-acting! he shouted.

She made him wicked because she needed someone who was wicked. She set her children against him. He became their enemy. So that Mummy could play at being what she wasn't, a good and protective mother.

The words rushed out of his mouth. He had nothing left to lose. He'd already made himself impossible a hundred times over. He picked up a heavy ashtray and threw it against the wall in the kitchen. A tile was broken. I can see where it happened. The rest of the tile is still there. They haven't bothered to replace it.

He rushed up to the room where Berit and I slept. He took hold of me and ran down the stairs. You and I, Asa, the two of us against them!

What are you doing? Mummy stood in his path before the front door. He pushed her aside. She tried to hold onto him. He struck off her hands.

He threw himself into the car, put me in the back seat and locked the doors so that Mummy couldn't get in. The car started with a roar.

He didn't look back. He drove out onto the motorway. He steered with his left hand and stretched back his right hand towards me in the back seat. He patted me.

It was over. An experiment in happiness had failed. He didn't know where he was going. In the state he was in he might have driven over a quay in the harbour.

§

He parked outside the Centre. He carried me under his arm as though I were a rag doll. He threw open the doors so they almost came off their hinges.

We've been tricked!

It was the physical therapist he was looking for. He marched into her office. His rage still gave him force.

You've tricked us. You and no one else.

I haven't tricked you.

Don't deny it! Don't lie to me. He spat out what he'd come to say. They'd put me through the exercises for nothing. The Method had been rejected.

By whom?

By those who know. By Science.

They stood on the floor in front of each other. Daddy still had me hanging under his right arm.

What Science are you talking about? the physical therapist asked him.

The doctors! The neurologists! The doctor from Prague is a bluff.

No!

You're using us as guinea pigs. Asa isn't going to get any better.

She will get better!

You've just been making use of us. Because of a whim in the mind of a mad doctor from Prague.

The physical therapist's nature, phlegmatic and abrupt, seemed to have changed. In fact she wasn't phlegmatic at all. It was just that she'd had difficulty expressing herself in Swedish. She wasn't abrupt. She was anything but abrupt.

A human being who flees must be borne by something. She was borne by fire and passion. In the middle of his rage Daddy noticed the transformation. She grew in stature in that dreary environment of fluorescent tubes and examination tables. Her fire was the kind of fire that can't be extinguished.

You think . . .

I know, Daddy interrupted her.

What is it you know?

This is what I know! Daddy confronted her with the article he'd read. See for yourself!

I've read it, she said.

Then you know it too. The doctor from Prague is a quack.

He's a genius, she said so quietly the words were almost soundless. She walked up to him and took me where I hung by his side. She took me and I didn't scream. It was strange.

He destroys children, Daddy said.

He helps them. Hundreds of children have been helped.

Then why is he rejected by Science?

Don't you understand . . . She carried me around in the room. She wasn't hard or brutal. She held me as though she were Mummy. Don't you understand that there's a conflict going on.

I know that, Daddy said. We fight everyday at home.

A scientific conflict, she said.

She told him about the scientific conflict while she rocked me on one arm. Once again he perceived her intensity. She talked about the new advances which were now being spread all over the world.

He wasn't listening any longer. He'd felt her fire. He saw how she held me and a new conviction grew inside him.

Only someone capable of love holds a child like that. It was the others, the other side, that he must seek out.

A small country, he'd written in his diary. Our country is a small country. A backyard in a corner of the world. The last country to be reached by the sun. An academic backyard, he's written, where people watch over their preserves and reward each other with titles. Someone was guilty. He was going to seek out whoever it was. Before this day was over he'd find out who was the cause of his suffering.

He went up to the physical therapist and took me from her.

You'll go on doing the exercises with Asa, she said.

He shrugged. He didn't think so. The possibilities weren't there anymore.

Do the exercises with her as before.

He was on his way towards the door.

You'll manage it, he heard her say behind him.

He didn't close the door. He didn't excuse himself for barging in. He walked straight out with me, the rag doll under his arm.

§

He was out in the poisoned stream of cars. He swung the car in and out of the lane, drove on the wrong side when the street was blocked, and rushed on with a burst of curses and blaring horns at his back.

He had no more than a vague idea of what he was going to do. It was some sort of revenge. How can one count the cost of losing what is most precious of all?

He skidded through a roundabout. The car engine howled at top speed. It was a crazy drive. He was on the north side of the city and pulled up in front of the big hospital. There was no parking space. He left the car on a pedestrian crossing.

He bent over the rear seat, took me in his arms and carried me in through the hospital doors. He was going to place me in front of Science. He knew that as, his face white, he rushed through long corridors. Take responsibility for what you've done! You destroyed our hopes. You cut off the last thread of life. Here she is, our spastic kid! Here she is on your shining desk. Take her and show what you can do.

You can't. You don't want to! But I tell you that you must. Isn't there room for her on your desk? Not even that. Your desk only has room for sarcasms about those of us who struggle and tear until our fingernails bleed.

Daddy caught sight of the senior physician's door. He stopped. Obscure intentions had driven him to this point. His mind was unclear. What he intended to do now was completely meaningless.

I've come to demand responsibility! I've come for revenge! What did that mean? He didn't know.

A woman in a white coat approached him.

Who are you looking for?

He didn't answer. He looked past her. The senior physician's door was open. He walked towards the door. Now, Asa! If we don't do it now it'll be too late. The woman in the white coat remained where she was. Something was wrong. Hesitantly she followed him.

Daddy had held me pressed against him. Now he took me in both hands. He held me in front of him and stood motionless on the threshold to the senior physician's room.

The senior physician sat in a wheelchair.

I can imagine that the situation took a maximum of 20 seconds. How can 20 seconds be stretched out to eternity? Daddy stood there with me on the threshold. The senior physician sat in his wheelchair, absorbed in his documents.

Daddy turned and walked away.

The woman in the white coat caught up with him. Did you want something?

I must have taken a wrong turning, Daddy muttered.

He walked through the corridors with a bitter taste in his mouth. What he had seen was a man so weak he could scarcely lift a sheet of paper. Daddy saw the senior physician's magazine article in front of him with its scornful declaration of war. The man in the wheelchair wanted the entire world in wheelchairs! Could that be it? Every child who dances and jumps is a defeat to someone who is crippled?

He thought about this while retracing his steps through the corridors. You don't have to believe in everything you think. I'm not sure that he really believed in the absurd declaration that said that the doctor in the wheelchair wanted to see all children in wheelchairs. But these thoughts brought new revelations.

He'd noticed the physical therapist's hands. She worked with her senses and her body as a violinist works when presenting the piece that will make him a master.

Daddy walked out through the hospital doorway. He and I!

It wasn't Science he had met. He thought he understood that now. He'd stood in front of a tragic doctor who could never lift the children, who could never feel and experience what was sick in them. A doctor who was forever cut off from the innermost secrets and so was obliged to combat what he had been cut off from. Those affected the most taking it upon themselves to torment others who suffer.

We were out in the open air. Daddy gave me wet kisses all over the face. He walked up to the car and discovered a parking ticket on the windscreen.

Good God, Asa! What have we done? This is crazy. The car was parked on a pedestrian crossing. They've given us a ticket!

§

I was one year old. My sister took clumsy little steps and rejoiced over her freedom.

They continued the exercises.

Don't ask me where they got their new conviction from. I don't know.

I was one year old and I still couldn't turn, sit or crawl.

I see the world gather around the floundering and screaming being that was me. I see Aunt Tilly and old Elsa. I see Science in his wheelchair.

I can hear how they condemn Mummy and Daddy. You fools! Haven't you learnt anything?

I spat blood. It happened when Daddy did the exercises with me and when I screamed more than usual. A blood vessel burst. It was in my throat or my mouth. Blood came out of my mouth.

Now, at any rate, now you must stop!

PART THREE

Chapter Thirteen

I lift up my rabbit from the wastepaper basket. It's all over now! You needn't be afraid any longer. I carry the rabbit to the windowsill. Morning is entering the city with huge jumps.

Here we stand, my rabbit and I. My window is a lookout post. My window is the victor's balcony.

My story left me when I was a year old. Imagine the next picture. It's five or six years later. Can you see what I see?

People are standing around on the lawn between the apple trees. Those who doubt have gathered. There's Aunt Tilly with her belief in destiny. That child will never be healthy. And Elsa with her tears that were always there because she had to hear my cries. Elsa is older now. But she's there.

Come closer! Step forward! A child whirls across the grass. What is she doing? How can anyone whirl round like that?

A child does cartwheels as though she were a little cloud of arms and legs.

Elsa stands with her mouth open and her poor-sighted eyes screwed up. Who is that kid doing cartwheels like that? A young gymnast, perhaps, or a Chinese monkey!

The cartwheeling child has one arm behind her back. Now you can see her clearly. She's doing cartwheels on one hand! Now you can see who the child is. It's me, Asa!

§

You don't believe it. Aunt Tilly will never believe it. She can believe some of it. That I got better. But this!

People don't set off out into the Milky Way. They just don't do it.

For Aunt Tilly and for many others I remained the spastic kid. That was why I wanted to show them. When, out in the country that summer, the other children began to do cartwheels I stood beside and watched. I tried to imitate them but I was clumsy and I fell.

God, how furious I got. I can do it! I'll show you!

I began to practice. I practiced all summer out in the country and when we moved back onto town I went on practicing. It got better. Soon I could do cartwheels on one hand. None of the other kids could do that.

When Mummy walked along the street I did cartwheels beside her. I did cartwheels on the platform when we waited for the underground train, and I did cartwheels between the tables when we went to cafés.

Granny came from far away. We hugged each other and we laughed. She cried and she laughed alternately. I knew it, she said. I knew it all the time.

That's what she's like, my fairytale Granny.

She knew and, from somewhere, my parents got back their conviction after the despairing days when I was one year old. How they did it remains a mystery to me.

Mummy cleaned out the refrigerator. It was full of pots and the pots were full of old food with green moss and disgusting hairy things. Daddy opened all the windows, he vacuum cleaned and scrubbed.

She promised never again to put her feet on the table at meals.

He promised to try to stop educating Patrick.

Then they went up to the bedroom and made love. They'd forgotten what it was like. It was like falling in love again, they say.

I got better. The big breakthrough had happened.

When I was fifteen months I could sit up. I began to turn over by myself.

But don't think I stopped screaming. I was the worst kid for screaming they'd ever had at the Centre.

The physical therapist was more straightforward now. I think she changed a little, too. She moderated the exercises and showed them more of her secrets. It was just she and they.

I got a new programme of exercises. I couldn't crawl and it was crawling I learnt during five long months. Finally I could do it. Sometimes I fell ill. Each time there was a break in the exercises I deteriorated.

Now only my hands were left. Precision motricity, Daddy's written. It was then they discontinued the exercises. They felt I'd done enough screaming.

It took a long time before I could use my hands. I couldn't pick up small things. The thumb and index finger are used for picking up things with, and mine wouldn't obey me.

I still write with my left hand. I'll always be a spastic kid, although almost no one notices it. In fact I'm right-handed. But most of the damage is on the right side. So I learnt to write with my left hand.

It's quite difficult. Try and you'll see for yourself.

When I started school I had to spend the first year in a class for physically disabled children. Most of the others were in wheelchairs. I could do cartwheels but I was still in pretty bad shape. I still found it difficult to use my hands. And I drew things backwards. I wrote letters backwards and upside down. Mummy says that's part of it. I couldn't care less. It was a phase and it passed.

Poor old Elsa had a terrible time. She came back to us for a while. She was so kind to us. But then the accident happened. She was in a lift with Putte. She couldn't see very well and when she entered the lift Putte's collar got caught in the outside of the lift door around the handle.

She pressed the button. Putte shot up to the ceiling in

front of her eyes and was strangled. Poor Elsa! She got worse. Soon she was almost blind.

They went to visit her at Christmas. I don't know where she is now.

Mummy gave up the Celestial Wardrobe. Most of all she wanted to be an architect. She wanted to furnish houses Aunt Tilly wouldn't be allowed into. She wanted everyone to be able to live in white rooms and sit on chairs that don't give you backache. But she didn't become an architect. Instead she does something artistic and I'm not quite sure what it is.

Daddy didn't go back to his old theater. He talks about the play he put on their table. That play! His face lights up. They couldn't decide. They were forced to put it on because they didn't have anything else. Fifty thousand people came to see it.

The actors made money, Daddy says. But in fact they thought the play was rubbish and they thought that those who liked it were rubbish as well. Afterwards they sought out a new audience and became respectable.

I think he's being ridiculous when he talks about it. It was such a long time ago. He becomes closed up and bitter. Besides, his old theater had several successes later on. Without him.

What we did was right, Asa. Wasn't what we did right?

They ask me. I know more now. I've travelled with them through that long night. I've been inside their hiding places and I think I've dug out every dream they had. And yet there's still something I can't get at.

That something! During quiet moments in Mummy's bed it seems close. Like gentle wingbeats. Friends who breathe and live. It seems so close when we've switched off the light and she holds her hand around mine.

I know that she wants to meet the doctor from Prague. He's no flight of fancy. He really exists and it was with him they joined forces. She thought of travelling to Munich where he lives. But nothing came of it.

When I lie in Mummy's bed I know that she's with those who try to reach the light. She hasn't changed. She wanted to give the doctor from Prague something just the same, an old debt she wants to pay off. His people, his tortured people. She puts money in collection boxes and pulls her conscience over me like a quilt when it's time for me to go to sleep.

Can it be her conscience? Can it be her conscience that gave her the courage to fight?

As far as the doctor from Prague is concerned, Daddy says, the lackeys there couldn't stand him. What's extraordinary, he says, is that the same thing happened here. There are those with the souls of lackeys here too, although they dress themselves out in gentle understanding.

It's Saturday morning. I've been awake all night and to my surprise I notice that I'm no longer tired. I'll go down to the kitchen and lay the table for them to make them happy. I long for Berit, my beloved twin. And I must pack my basketball gear. Our basketball team has a tournament that begins at ten o'clock.

What we did was right, wasn't it, Asa?

Yes, I say. You did what was right. You did what you had to do.

Although, of course, I couldn't know. I've said that before. Who am I to judge what's medically right? According to the doctors here what they did was wrong. According to them I should now be a mental wreck after the torments I've been subjected to.

I remember the doctor with the French name. I met him when I was discharged from the Centre. He examined me and I did cartwheels for him.

There you see, he said. Just as I suspected from the beginning. All those exercises were unnecessary. You can see for yourselves. Asa is healthy!

Actually, I don't care about all that. It's the basketball match that's important now.

PART FOUR

The Author Discusses the Vojta Method

At the end of the 1960s, a new method of treatment by remedial exercises for children with cerebral palsy was introduced in Sweden. The originator of this method was the Czechoslovakian neurologist Vaclav Vojta. His method was introduced by leading physiotherapists who felt that they had made a breakthrough. Hundreds of children began to be treated by what came to be called the Vojta Method.

Most of the medical profession reacted quite differently. Their condemnation of the Vojta exercises was almost unanimous. It was said, firstly, to be unscientific, and, secondly, said its critics, there was a risk of causing mental harm to the children.

Such violent reaction led to the desired result. Parents were warned against the method. Even among physiotherapists, there were many whose enthusiasm cooled.

By the middle of the 1970s, treatment by the strictly applied Vojta system of exercises had disappeared almost entirely.

Rightly or wrongly?

Sweden is a comparatively small country on the medical map of the world. Very few doctors have specialized in child neurology. There were, in reality, two or three leading specialists who were active in changing the general opinion.

Their criticism was aimed at parts of Doctor Vojta's reasoning which they felt they had proved to be far too sweeping and ill-founded. "Vojta is a bluff," was the conclusion expounded in the medical journals.

The opinion of its supporters is that the critics never really acquainted themselves with the Vojta method. It can be difficult to change one's thinking when old and tried conceptions are suddenly rejected. For example, it was earlier considered good for a child with cerebral palsy injuries to stand as soon as possible—at all costs—even those who could not stand alone. They were provided with splints and supports to get them up. And then Vojta comes along and says that this is absolutely forbidden because it will cause the manifestation of all the pathological movements. Down on the floor with the children instead. Let them crawl!

Belief or scientific fact?

Vojta feels his method make it possible to break through the blockages suffered by children with cerebral palsy. In order to prove this, it is necessary to conduct comparative studies. A certain number of children should be exercised and a corresponding number left without treatment. Dr. Vojta himself has rejected such research. In his opinion, it is unethical. All children should receive treatment if they are believed to be injured.

Then, in the early 1980s, a comparative study was carried out in Sweden. Twenty children suffering from cerebral palsy were chosen. Lots were drawn and one group treated by the Vojta method and another by the English Bobath method.

There were in both groups children whose injuries were so severe that improvement by physiotherapy was considered almost impossible. Among the other children, it was found that three of six children treated by the Bobath method recovered completely, while eight of nine children treated by the Vojta method recovered completely. This should be an indication that Vojta's method is superior. But the study was considered insufficient because there were too few children in the test.

Though Sweden said no to Vojta, there are one or two physiotherapists in Sweden still persevering in utilizing his method. In other countries, the reaction was quite the opposite. There, Doctor Vojta is regarded as an important neurologist. His method is practiced, particularly in West Germany and in Japan.

There is a report from Japan regarding a study (described in *Medicine and Child Neurology* no. 26, 1984). Two groups of children with cerebral palsy injuries were compared. One group—children with severe injuries—was treated at an early stage by the Vojta system of exercises. In the other group—children with less severe injuries—treatment by the Vojta method began later. The children's injuries were verified by so-called computer-tomography findings.

The results after treatment were important. The severely injured children—that is to say those who were given early treatment—learned to sit up later, it is true, than the slightly injured (on the average at the age of 19.8 months as opposed to 15.2 months). Nevertheless, the seriously injured group learned to crawl at an earlier age than the other group (12 to 15 months). And they started to walk at twenty-two months, whereas the slightly injured children first began to walk at the age of thirty months. So, through the Vojta method, the severely injured children caught up developmentally with the slightly injured. That is the unequivocal finding of the Japanese study.

By early treatment of, for example, spastic diplegia, cerebral palsy can be avoided. Without treatment, these children develop cerebral palsy injuries.

Belief or knowledge?

Again, Sweden said no to Vojta. What is considered scientific in Germany and Japan was pronounced unscientific in Sweden.

As you have read earlier in this book, Asa screamed

while she was undergoing treatment. According to the Swedish specialists, she was being exposed to incalculable mental injury through these exercises. The opinion that children using the Vojta method were subjected to emotional harm became predominant among members of the medical profession in Sweden and is even prevalent today.

Of course, as Asa's parents, we have often wondered whether the treatment has caused her any emotional disturbance. Such thoughts are almost always close at hand after a period of struggle and despair. But we are unable to confirm the fears of the doctors.

In a symposium at a medical congress in Stockholm in November, 1985, a study of the mental reactions—both of the parents of children with cerebral palsy injuries and of the children themselves—was presented. The study constitutes the latest part of the report on the project referred to above, where children treated respectively by the Vojta or the Bobath method were tested and compared.

This study does not support the severe criticism of the Vojta method. It became evident that nearly all small children feel discomfort when they undergo physiotherapy. All the children being treated by the Vojta method screamed under treatment. Eight of the thirteen children undergoing Bobath treatment screamed.

The parents also experienced great difficulties. Several parents in the Vojta group appeared to have greater difficulty in managing their reactions during the period of treatment. The parents in the Bobath group felt the strain of treatment being carried out both day and night and through all the children's activities. In both groups, there were many parents who were afraid of doing something wrong which could further injure their children.

How did the children develop later? This is, of course, the main question. The critics are of the opinion that the children treated by the Vojta method had their mental health almost ruined. This was not the case. None of the

Vojta-treated children afterwards showed any signs of emotional disturbance whatsoever, according to their parents. Of the thirteen Bobath-treated children, however, there were four who showed slight or moderate signs of emotional disability.

It should be noted that this study was carried out with what we call soft data. One unfortunate conclusion which may be drawn is that the Vojta system of exercises can be tougher on both children and parents. On the other hand, however, more of the Vojta-treated children were in better mental shape afterwards. The explanation for this could be that almost all the Vojta-treated children recovered completely.

SOME QUESTIONS AND ANSWERS

Here are some notes taken of a talk I had with a doctor who had familiarized himself with Doctor Vojta's method of treatment.

Q. Who is Doctor Vojta?

A. He is a Czechoslovakian neurologist. He has analyzed patterns of human movement and the divergences that can be observed. He did most of his work in Czechoslovakia. He fled from there in 1968 and his ideas have since spread to the West.

Q. I suppose there are other forms of remedial exercises for physically disabled children?

A. Yes, various methods have been developed, for instance, by the Bobaths and by Lewitt in England, by Doman-Delacato in the United States and by Doctor Peto in Hungary. In Sweden, more recently, another method has been developed by Helga Hirschfeld.

Q. At the time of Asa's treatment, is it not true that most physiotherapists were using the Bobath method?

A. Yes. The Bobaths are an English couple: she a physiotherapist and he a doctor. They have devoted their lives to children with cerebral palsy. Some parts of the treatment are the same in both the Vojta and Bobath methods. In both cases, an attempt is made to diagnose the pattern of the child's movements and to start treatment at the existing level. Bobath examines the pathological reflexes and tries to impede them.

Q. Vojta chose another way, didn't he?

A. That is correct. His method does not involve blocking.

Q. What is the method, then?

A. Let me give you a picture. In the spinal cord, there is a program of movement-patterns remaining from the period in man's evolution when he was still an animal. Crawling is the natural movement of a reptile. When you observe a crocodile, you see that its arms and legs are outspread and it moves by crawling. Animals, a little higher on the evolutionary scale, creep with all their extremities drawn in under their bodies. All these programs are stored at higher or lower levels, from the spinal cord and upwards. The child with cerebral palsy cannot reach the cortex—that is, the level of the cerebral cortex—and, by its own will, make the necessary movements. There is some injury in the way. There is a system of tracks leading from the cortex down to the spinal cord and out to the muscles. Somewhere in the system, damage has occurred. That is the reason why the child cannot, by its own will, carry out certain movements. However, the child still has the programed pattern of movement at a lower level. Vojta makes use of this pattern of movement. If the child can be induced to use it, it is possible—in Vojta's opinion—to teach the child to perform movements it is unable at first to perform by its own will. After which, hopefully, new tracking from the outside in will be established. This can be done as long as the nervous system is developing.

Q. Then exercising has to begin early?

A. The nervous system develops a great deal during the first year. The younger the child, the less mature is the nervous system. It is a question of using to advantage its period of development. Above all, it is important to use the primitive movements, which is what happens in the case of reflex crawling itself. By making use of this level, the child can be induced to bend and stretch all its extremities and the whole body can be made to coordinate these movements in a primitive pattern of movement.

Q. Must it be done against the child's will?

A. Yes. The child cannot bend its extremities when it is a question of control by will. Then, for example, fear takes over the reflexes so that the child can stretch, but not bend.

Q. One forces the child?

A. Yes. The child must be forced to use its reflexes for creeping, something it cannot do spontaneously. He or she must be provoked into it. The child is placed in a certain position, a crawling position. The child is held fast in that position. In that way, a forward movement is induced by making use of the so-called reflex zones in the extremities and the trunk. The reflexes in the spinal cord are made use of. Such reflexes express themselves even among adults, for example, when they are struck on the knee. A reflex signal goes inward to the spinal cord and is answered, as everyone knows, by a sudden jerk of the leg. It is something of the same thing, although in this case the pattern of reflexes is rather more complicated, as the whole body and all the extremities are involved. One can also build up muscular response and hope in that way to establish a new pathway from the periphery in towards the cerebral cortex. Let me give you another example. If we don't use our eyes, the part of the cortex which has to do with sight does not develop. It needs to be in continual use, with pathways coming in from outside, in order to develop. In a similar way, the part of the cortex concerned with movement is assisted by the Vojta treatment to give an answer and a correct pattern of movement.

Q. But forcing? Asa was provoked terribly. Is it right to force a little child?

A. Yes, it is right. By holding the child fast, we force her or him to carry out movements which they find very difficult. But it doesn't hurt; it is not painful.

To those who were not familiar with it—particularly doctors—the Vojta method seemed terrible. One forces the child and the child is unhappy. My opinion is that Sweden is probably not the right country in which to introduce this kind of treatment. People here are not used to authoritative treatment.

The Vojta treatment was started at the same time as a particularly gentle manner towards children, in all circumstances, at day-nursery and everywhere, was advocated. Suddenly, here was a method of treatment that involved making children do what they didn't want to do.

This is certainly a great difference if one compares Sweden with a country like Japan, where children are successfully treated by the Vojta method. Japanese children continually have to do things they don't wish to do or dislike doing. It is part of their pattern of life. Applying the Vojta technique, Japanese parents probably do not experience the same difficulty in forcing their children to do something which they believe is for the good of the child.

Q. What does Vojta himself say?

A. He says he has never known any child to suffer mental harm from the treatment. Besides, there is so much to be gained from the fact that the children get well physically.

Q. What injuries does the Vojta method not help against?

A. According to Vojta, it does not help in the most severe cases—those of massive changes in the brain. One cannot compensate for the absence of brain tissue.

Q. According to the critics, quite a number of children are treated unnecessarily with the help of Vojta's positionary reflexes. According to them, many children would have got better in any case.

A. There are certainly some children who are treated unnecessarily by the Vojta Method. Vojta himself probably treats numerous children unnecessarily. The question is, "Is it worth it?" Perhaps it is, when we know that at the same time many children are being saved.

Right or wrong? Asa was treated for a period of a year—an arduous year. Was it all unnecessary?

§

The physiotherapist responsible for the therapy remembers Asa. I asked him to explain what was wrong with Asa.

A. She lacked postural firmness.

Q. What does that mean?

A. It means basic posture. The child must be able to lie on its stomach and on its back and be in control. She couldn't. She had no stability in any position at all. She was controlled by reflexes. I remember it very well.

The diagnosis was tonus fluctuation, that is to say either very slack or enormously tense.

She was slack when lying down. Her muscular tension was too low. But when we started working on her, she tensed herself enormously. It was difficult. We had to hold her very firmly and she reacted correspondingly.

Q. Her feet were stretched to a point and her head strained backwards?

A. That is typical. We call it the opisthotonic position. The muscles of her back were enormously stretched and she lacked corresponding firmness of the muscles on the other side. This was how such great tensions arose.

Q. What is meant by "tonus"?

A. Muscular tonus is the tension in muscles that everybody has. Normal tonus is what gives us a certain posture. We can perform certain coordinated movements. Children who sustain brain-damage have their tonus impaired by the injury to the brain. It can become either too high or too low. The problem was to get the muscles to coordinate so that the tonus became normal.

Q. When the child is so little, it must be a question of involuntary reflexes?

A. The reflexes spoken of here are those which will disappear from the clinical picture by the time the child is six months or one year old. These primitive reflexes will disappear then. The child will then begin to coordinate and use its will more and more. But in the cases of children with brain damage, these reflexes do not disappear. They remain evident. Motor coordination remains at a very primitive level. At the level of four to six weeks of age. The child gradually begins to use its will to move. Then the child cannot use the normal movements, but is forced to use the abnormal. This creates a vicious circle. If help is not forthcoming, things will only go from bad to worse. We call this the development of pathological movement.

Normally, children begin to rotate their arms in outward movements, while the primitive reflex movements are all inward. Rotation inward of both shoulders and legs increases more and more. In this way, the pathological image is strengthened and becomes fixed.

Q. Asa held her thumb inside her hand; is this part of inward rotation?
A. Yes, it's a part of it. When the primitive reflexes disappear, the hand ceases to be clenched so tightly and begins to open.
Q. When does this happen?
A. At about four, five, six months of age. It develops, but does not happen at once. The child's dexterity improves all the time. The tonus of the gripping reflex can last up to six months. The motor coordination of the hand develops most between the age of six and nine months.
Q. When should a child be able to turn over?
A. The ability to turn develops between the ages of three and six months. At six months the child turns over and gets up on its knees.
Q. Is that the first advanced movement the child makes?
A. Not quite, but it's the first propelling movement. If the child can coordinate sufficiently to turn over, it can also coordinate sufficiently to be able to creep. It is important that the child manages to turn over in the right way.
Q. What is the next step in the child's development?
A. Just a minute. We must first observe how it lies on its stomach. The child manages this at about three, four months. It is then stable. Then the child supports itself on its elbows and can thus free its head

from the movements of its arms. At first, the head can only move in connection with the arm movements. Now the child stabilizes itself on both its elbows and can turn its head freely. This is the first important point in the physical development of the child. After that it can turn over. It is at the age of six months, the child turns over. Between the ages of six and nine months, the child practices turning over and stabilizing itself on its knees and gradually begins to move forward on its knees. At first its creeping movements are immature and clumsy, but become gradually more and more coordinated. At ten months, the child is creeping really well.

Q. Turning over is a very advanced operation, isn't it? How is it done?

A. The child has to bend its legs to turn over. And lift its pelvis. This is a very important movement that the child practices for several months. We can observe this when the child plays with its feet. Not only is it important to the child to feel its feet, the child lifting its pelvis also contributes to stabilizing the trunk.

Children who develop abnormally cannot do this. Some children with cerebral palsy can perhaps bend their legs, that is to say those whose tonus is not too high, but they cannot lift the pelvis. This is a difficult and complicated movement.

In turning, the child also lifts its pelvis. In the next phase, the child begins to twist its body and, in that phase, the movements of the legs are differentiated. This differentiation is very important.

Children with these kind of injuries can sometimes bend their legs, but are not able to carry out differentiated leg-movements. We call this turning "en bloc." These children continue to turn "en bloc" all the time. They bend both legs and throw themselves round in some way.

Q. What is meant by lifting the pelvis?

A. The upper part of the body acts as a stabilizer. For example, when a child puts its feet into its mouth the pelvis is pulled up high. When turning, one arm is stretched and the child stabilizes itself on one shoulder when the trunk rotates. When turning to the right, the right leg is stretched at the same time as the left leg is bent.

Q. How would Asa have developed without treatment?

A. As Asa's reflexes were very defective, she would have developed tonus fluctuation. A child with such a disability gradually becomes quite stiff and can never get up on all fours. All turning is done by stretching and, finally, the child becomes fixed in its stretching movements. This is a very tragic prospect. Asa's development was heading that way. My experience leads me to that conclusion, but it is impossible to prove.

Q. How did the Vojta method develop in Czechoslovakia?

A. It developed during the sixties. Vojta was a neurologist at the children's department of the neurological clinic in Prague. Many people brought their children there. He began to study the motor coordination of the children. He found that the older children with injuries moved in exactly the same way as newborn children. He discovered that their development was arrested. It was his theory that this was not the result of any disease; development was arrested and it was a question of blocking.

The primitive movements are the ones that endure. One has to force a way into the normal muscular coordination and, in that way, attempt to by-pass the brain-damage to enable other parts of the brain to take over.

In this way, Vojta discovered an opportunity for us. If we can manage to break through the blocking, we can get normal movements going.

Q. So the exercises facilitate the use of parts of the brain other than those damaged?

A. This, in itself, was not only Volta's idea. There are many who have engaged in research in the field of neurology. They have also reached the conclusion that compensation in the brain is something that exists.

Q. But the Vojta Method proposed something new, didn't it?

A. Yes. Managing to find how to exercise a little mite effectively was really a fantastic achievement. Of course, the child can be stimulated—toys are given to the child and the child takes them. But, in doing this, we stimulate the child to use the movements of which it is capable—that is to say we stimulate the child into even more use of the erroneous pattern of movement. Although we try to guide its movements, that will be the result. In the brain, too.

Q. Have you had a lot of successes?

A. Many children have gotten well. But I cannot prove scientifically that they would not have recovered without remedial exercises.

Q. But in Japan they consider that they have proof?

A. Yes. We carried out a comparative study in Sweden. But the results were not accepted as they rested on too small a basis.

Q. Doctor Vojta makes use of what are called the positionary reflexes to diagnose infants. According to a rather recent Swedish study, almost half of all healthy children show aberrancies. Is this not a rejection of Doctor Vojta's method of diagnosis?

A. Vojta has never claimed that positionary reflexes are sufficient for an early diagnosis. Postural firmness is the basis and the other is complementary.

One cannot diagnose cerebral palsy injuries in a child showing aberrancies at the age of four months. One can only establish that there are certain disorders and that treatment can be necessary. Such treatment will soon show whether the child is developing well and will recover.

Still, an experienced neurologist or physiotherapist does not often make mistakes.

Q. But is there a risk of unnecessary treatment?

A. I myself have examined healthy children in Alby and it appeared that some of them had faulty positionary reflexes at the age of three months. There could have been four or five children with faulty reflexes.

The important thing is to do follow-up studies on these children. Those whose faulty reflexes increase are most often those who need treatment. The fact is that if a healthy child who is only a little under-stimulated is given treatment, the resulting improvement will be so unbelievably speedy that the treatment can be terminated after as little as two to eight weeks.

But those who are not familiar with the method do not realize this. They think that we sometimes spend a year or two treating a child who does not need treatment. This is not the case.

Q. Surely you have had some failures?

A. Many years ago, there were occasions when my great enthusiasm about the treatment led me to misjudge a child's possibilities. I raised too high hopes and that led to disappointment.

Q. What does Doctor Vojta look like?

A. Not thin, not fat. Sturdy. Not very tall, enormously charming, enormously vital. Not much hair on his head. Warm, brown eyes.

Q. Can you describe Doctor Vojta?

A. He's a very special person, a genius.

Q. What do you mean by special?

A. He is very warm-hearted. He cares about the children and their parents. He is very well liked. He gives parents the feeling of security they are looking for in their doctor. He explains things in detail to them and is very conscientious. He draws up very tangible small projects and parts of projects which parents are really able to carry out. I, too, try to work in the same way. To talk to the parents about what will happen in a month or two. Having projects divided into small parts is very important to parents; being able to look forward to some slight progress, the child beginning to grip, for instance.

Of course, as her father I ask myself, was it right or wrong to treat Asa.

One cannot be certain. Not one-hundred percent. However, there is strong reason to believe that there would have been no basketball match for Asa if we—her parents—had followed the advice of the other doctors and refrained from the Vojta exercises. Asa would probably be sitting in a wheelchair now.